Single Best Answer MCQs in

ANAESTHESIA

Volume I Clinical Anaesthesia

Cyprian Mendonca, Mahesh Chaudhari, Josephine James

tfm Publishing Limited, Castle Hill Barns, Harley, Nr Shrewsbury, SY5 6LX, UK. Tel: +44 (0)1952 510061; Fax: +44 (0)1952 510192 E-mail: nikki@tfmpublishing.com; Web site: www.tfmpublishing.com

Design & Typesetting: Nikki Bramhill BSc Hons Dip Law
First Edition: © September 2010
Background cover image © Comstock Inc., www.comstock.com

ISBN: 978 1 903378 75 5

ii

Printed by Gutenberg Press Ltd., Gudja Road, Tarxien, PLA 19, Malta. Tel: +356 21897037; Fax: +356 21800069.

Contents

Preface

Single best answer type multiple choice questions are being introduced into anaesthetic postgraduate examinations. They are considered to be a valuable way of assessing the trainee's ability to apply knowledge to clinical practice.

This book consists of six sets of single best answer practice papers. Each set comprises 30 multiple choice questions drawn from clinical anaesthesia, pain and intensive care medicine. Each question consists of a stem describing a clinical scenario or problem followed by five possible answer options. One of them is the best response for the given question. Each question and answer is accompanied by supporting notes obtained from peer-reviewed journal articles and anaesthesia textbooks.

The main objective of this book is to provide trainees with a series of single best answer type questions that will prepare them for this format of postgraduate examinations. Much emphasis has been placed on the application of knowledge to solve common peri-operative problems encountered during anaesthetic practice.

We hope that a thorough revision of this book will enable trainees to improve their ability to apply knowledge to clinical practice. We believe this book will not only be an invaluable educational resource for those who are preparing for postgraduate examinations, but will also be of benefit to any practising anaesthetist.

Cyprian Mendonca MD, FRCA
Consultant Anaesthetist
University Hospitals Coventry and Warwickshire
Coventry, UK

Mahesh Chaudhari MD, FRCA, FFPMRCA
Consultant Anaesthetist
Worcestershire Royal Hospital
Worcester, UK

Josephine James FRCA
Consultant Anaesthetist
Heart of England Foundation Trust
Birmingham, UK

v

Acknowledgements

We are grateful to Nikki Bramhill, Director, tfm publishing, for critically reviewing the manuscript. We extend our thanks to the following who contributed questions to this book:

Dr Thejas Bhari
Specialty Registrar, Warwickshire School of Anaesthesia

Dr Thomas Billyard
Specialty Registrar, Warwickshire School of Anaesthesia

Dr Narotham Burri
Specialty Registrar, Warwickshire School of Anaesthesia

Dr Shefali Chaudhari
Specialty Registrar, Warwickshire School of Anaesthesia

Dr Adrian Jennings
Specialty Registrar, Birmingham School of Anaesthesia

Dr Payal Kajekar
Specialty Registrar, Warwickshire School of Anaesthesia

Dr Seema Quasim
Consultant Anaesthetist, University Hospital, Coventry

Dr Mohan Ranganathan
Consultant Anaesthetist, George Eliot Hospital, Nuneaton

Dr Rajneesh Sachdeva
Specialty Registrar, Warwickshire School of Anaesthesia

Dr Rathinavel Shanmugam
Specialty Registrar, Warwickshire School of Anaesthesia

Dr Catherine Snaith
Specialty Registrar, Warwickshire School of Anaesthesia

Dr Joyce Yeung
Specialty Registrar, Warwickshire School of Anaesthesia

Abbreviations

AAA	Abdominal aortic aneurysm
ACTH	Adrenocorticotrophic hormone
ADH	Anti-diuretic hormone
AF	Atrial fibrillation
AICD	Automatic implantable cardioverter defibrillator
ALS	Advanced life support
ALT	Alanine transaminase
APACHE	Acute Physiology and Chronic Health Evaluation
APTT	Activated partial thromboplastin time
ARDS	Acute respiratory distress syndrome
ASA	American Society of Anesthesiologists
ASAS	Anterior spinal artery syndrome
AST	Aspartate transaminase
BD	Twice a day
BE	Base excess
BJR	Bezold-Jarisch reflex
BP	Blood pressure
CABG	Coronary artery bypass grafting
CAP	Community-acquired pneumonia
CBT	Cognitive behavioural therapy
CEA	Carotid endarterectomy
CK	Creatine kinase
Cl	Chloride
CNS	Central nervous system
CO	Carbon monoxide
COAD	Chronic obstructive airway disease
COHb	Carboxy-haemoglobin

COPD	Chronic obstructive pulmonary disease
CPAP	Continuous positive airway pressure
CPM	Central pontine myelinolysis
CPR	Cardiopulmonary resuscitation
CPSP	Chronic post-surgical pain
CRPS	Complex regional pain syndrome
CSE	Combined spinal epidural
CSF	Cerebrospinal fluid
CSWS	Cerebral salt wasting syndrome
CT	Computed tomography
CVA	Cerebrovascular accident
CVP	Central venous pressure
DDAVP	1-de-amino-8-D-arginine vasopressin
DI	Diabetes insipidus
DIC	Disseminated intravascular coagulation
DKA	Diabetic ketoacidosis
DLCO	Diffusion lung capacity for carbon monoxide
DPG	2,3-diphosphoglycerate
DVT	Deep vein thrombosis
ECG	Electrocardiogram
EEG	Electro-encephalography
EMG	Electromyography
EMI	Electromagnetic interference
ESR	Erythrocyte sedimentation rate
$ETCO_2$	End-tidal CO_2
FDP	Fibrin degradation product
FEV	Forced expiratory volume
FFP	Fresh frozen plasma
FRC	Functional residual capacity
FVC	Forced vital capacity
GA	General anaesthesia
GABA	Gamma aminobutyric acid
GCS	Glasgow Coma Scale
GFR	Glomerular filtration rate
GH	Growth hormone
GTN	Glyceryl trinitrate
H	Hydrogen

Hb	Haemoglobin
HCO_3	Bicarbonates
Hct	Haematocrit
HDU	High dependency unit
HELLP	Haemolysis, elevated liver enzymes and low platelets
HIT	Heparin-induced thrombocytopaenia
ICP	Intracranial pressure
ICU	Intensive care unit
IDDS	Implantable drug delivery system
INR	International normalised ratio
IPH	Idiopathic pulmonary hypertension
ISS	Injury Severity Score
IV	Intravenous
JVP	Jugular venous pressure/pulse
K	Potassium
LA	Local anaesthesia
LBP	Low back pain
LMA	Laryngeal mask airway
LMWH	Low-molecular-weight heparin
MAOI	Monoamine oxidase inhibitor
MEP	Motor evoked potentials
MH	Malignant hyperthermia
MND	Motor neurone disease
MODS	Multiple Organ Dysfunction Score
MRA	Magnetic resonance angiography
MST	Morphine sulphate
Na	Sodium
NG	Nasogastric
NIBP	Non-invasive blood pressure
NICE	National Institute for Health and Clinical Excellence
NIDDM	Non-insulin dependent diabetes mellitus
NIV	Non-invasive ventilation
NMDA	N-methyl-D-aspartate
NPPE	Negative pressure pulmonary oedema
NSAID	Non-steroidal anti-inflammatory drug
OD	Once a day
OSF	Organ system failure

PCA	Patient-controlled analgesia
PCWP	Pulmonary capillary wedge pressure
PE	Pulmonary embolism
PEEP	Positive end expiratory pressure
PEFR	Peak expiratory flow rate
PHN	Post-herpetic neuralgia
POD	Postoperative delirium
PONV	Postoperative nausea and vomiting
PPH	Postpartum haemorrhage
PT	Prothrombin time
PTH	Parathyroid hormone
RBC	Red blood cell
RV	Residual volume
SAH	Subarachnoid haemorrhage
SAPS	Simplified Acute Physiology Score
SCD	Sickle cell disease
SCS	Spinal cord stimulator
SIADH	Syndrome of inappropriate anti-diuretic hormone secretion
SLE	Systemic lupus erythematosus
SOFA	Sequential organ failure assessment
SSEP	Somatosensory evoked potentials
SVC	Superior vena cava
SVR	Systemic vascular resistance
TDS	Three times a day
TENS	Transcutaneous electrical nerve stimulation
TFPI	Tissue factor prothrombin inhibitor
THAM	Tri-hydroxymethyl aminomethane
TIVA	Total intravenous anaesthesia
TLC	Total lung capacity
TLCO	Transfer factor for carbon monoxide
TRALI	Transfusion-related acute lung injury
TRH	Thyrotropin releasing hormone
TSH	Thyroid stimulating hormone
UFH	Unfractionated heparin
VA	Alveolar volume
VAE	Venous air embolism
VAS	Visual Analogue Score

VF	Ventricular fibrillation
VIP	Vasoactive intestinal peptide
VTE	Venous thrombo-embolism
WBC	White blood cell
WCC	White cell count

Set 1 questions

1   A 60-year-old male patient is admitted to the emergency department. He was working on his car in a garage and was found unconscious by his wife, with the garage door almost shut and the car engine running. On assessment, his GCS is 7, oxygen saturation is 99% and mucous membranes are 'cherry red' in colour. Which of the following actions is most appropriate in the immediate management?

a.   Take a full history from his wife to confirm the facts.
b.   Arrange for a CT of the brain to precisely diagnose the cause of unconsciousness.
c.   Arrange for urgent transfer to a neuro-intensive care unit.
d.   Intubate and ventilate the patient with 100% oxygen.
e.   Oxygenate with a non-rebreathing mask whilst arterial blood gas results are performed.

2   A 59-year-old male has undergone a left upper lobectomy for a neoplasm. The peri-operative course was uncomplicated. He has a history of COPD and 50-pack-per-year history of smoking. His routine medications include a salbutamol inhaler and uniphyllin 300mg b.d. On the second postoperative day, in the high dependency unit, the patient suddenly develops atrial fibrillation with a ventricular rate of 140 to 170 beats/min. His blood pressure falls

to 80/30mmHg from a near normal level for his age. The most appropriate immediate management is:

a.   Check the serum K⁺ and Mg⁺ levels.
b.   Commence oxygen 6L/min using a non-rebreathing mask.
c.   Give amiodarone 5mg/kg boluses over 30 minutes.
d.   Synchronised DC shock.
e.   Intravenous digoxin.

+3   A 21-year-old male has had an extraction of an impacted third molar tooth under general anaesthetic. Postoperatively he continues to bleed from the surgical site. Despite surgical exploration and packing, bleeding continues. His coagulation screen reveals both a prolonged bleeding time and activated partial thromboplastin time (APTT), but the prothrombin time (PT) and platelet count are within normal limits. The patient mentions that his father bruises quite easily. The most likely diagnosis is:

a.   Haemophilia A.
b.   Haemolytic uraemic syndrome.
c.   Haemophilia B.
d.   von Willebrand's disease.
e.   Laden V deficiency.

- 4   A 45-year-old man with a history of gall stones presents to the emergency department complaining of severe constant epigastric pain radiating to the back and flanks, and vomiting. Examination reveals pyrexia, abdominal distension, rebound tenderness and discolouration of the flanks. Which of the following blood tests would be most useful in the diagnosis of acute pancreatitis?

a.   Serum amylase.
b.   Serum trypsinogen.
c.   Serum lipase.
d.   Serum transaminases.
e.   Serum calcium.

*5 A 39-year-old male is due to undergo haemorrhoidectomy. He suffered a complete spinal cord transection at T6 level 2 years ago. His medications include paracetamol q.d.s., gabapentin 600mg t.d.s., omeprazole and clonazepam. He intermittently uses a GTN spray for the management of symptoms related to autonomic hyper-reflexia. The patient has no particular preference regarding anaesthetic technique. Which anaesthetic technique would be most suitable?

a. General anaesthesia with rapid sequence induction.
b. Spinal anaesthesia.
c. No need for any anaesthesia.
d. Light general anaethesia.
e. Combined spinal epidural (CSE).

6 An 83-year-old female presents to the pain clinic with a 10-week history of severe pain in her left eye. The pain is continuous and is associated with a burning sensation. She also had a skin rash in the painful area which began after a week of onset of the pain. She has been treated with an intermittent course of steroid medication for the management of her poorly controlled COAD. The most likely cause of her pain is:

a. Trigeminal neuralgia.
b. Atypical facial pain.
c. Atypical presentation of trigeminal neuralgia.
d. Late signs and symptoms of polymyalgia rheumatica.
e. Post-herpetic neuralgia.

*7 A 33-year-old female is due to undergo an emergency laparotomy for a ruptured ectopic pregnancy. She has had a previous general anaesthesic when she was told she might suffer from a possible allergy to an anaesthetic agent. She suffers from hay fever and has a history of allergic reactions to multiple medications including

3

antibiotics and NSAIDs. Her previous anaesthetic notes are not available. Which one of the following is most appropriate for intravenous induction of anaesthesia?

a.   Thiopentone.
b.   Propofol.
c.   Etomidate.
d.   Ketamine.
e.   Methohexitone.

 A 60-year-old male is undergoing elective posterior fossa surgery in the sitting position. Forty minutes into the operation, he develops bronchospasm and his blood pressure drops suddenly from 110/70mmHg to 70/40 mmHg. In the previous 20 minutes the patient had not received any drugs. What is the most likely cause of the sudden fall in BP in this patient?

a.   Myocardial infarction.
b.   High concentration of volatile agents.
c.   Profuse bleeding.
d.   Air embolism.
e.   Anaphylaxis.

 You are called to assess a 25-year-old female with a history of acute bilateral symmetrical descending paralysis. She has no changes in her mental status or sensory deficit, and is afebrile. Which of the following investigations will best help you to arrive at the diagnosis?

a.   Analysis of blood or stool for botulinum toxin.
b.   Blood culture for viruses.
c.   'Tensilon' test.
d.   CSF examination.
e.   Nerve conduction studies.

−10 A 61-year-old female is ready to be discharged on the fifth postoperative day following an uneventful total hip replacement. A nurse has noticed localised necrosis of skin at the sites of subcutaneous injection of enoxaparin on the abdominal wall. She also mentions that there has been a fall in platelet count from 216 x 10^9/L to 64 x 10^9/L over the last 5 days. What would be your next action?

a. Reduce the dose of enoxaparin by half and administer two units of FFP.
b. Stop enoxaparin.
c. Stop enoxaparin until the platelet count starts rising.
d. Stop enoxaparin and start an alternative anticoagulant.
e. Stop enoxaparin and transfuse two units of adult platelets.

⋆11 A 27-year-old woman has been diagnosed with untreatable carcinoma of the cervix and has severe pain. She is taking MST 400mg b.d., Oramorph 20mg four-hourly, gabapentin 600mg t.d.s. and clonazepam. The doses of opioid medication required to alleviate the pain have doubled in the last 2 months and the MST was changed to oxycodone and the dose increased, but with little effect on the degree of pain. Following palliative surgery she is now incontinent. Her life expectancy is about 3 months. The next best possible intervention for the management of her uncontrollable pain in the perineal area would be:

a. Radiofrequency lesioning of the lumbar sympathetic nerves.
b. Coeliac plexus block using a neurolytic solution.
c. Intrathecal saddle neurolytic block.
d. Intrathecal drug delivery of morphine.
e. Lumbar chemical sympathectomy using a neurolytic solution.

12 A 41-year-old primigravida has been admitted at 38 weeks of gestation with headache, nausea and a blood pressure of

196/116mmHg. A Caesarean section is planned, and oral labetalol 400mg has been administered. The next BP recorded an hour later is 176/110 mmHg. The next step in the control of this woman's pre-eclampsia should be:

a. Intravenous labetalol infusion.
b. Intravenous magnesium sulphate infusion, following a loading dose.
c. Intravenous magnesium sulphate infusion, without a loading dose.
d. Sublingual nifedipine tablet.
e. Epidural analgesia.

13 A 29-year-old woman (gravida 2, para 1) has had a ventouse vaginal delivery of a baby boy weighing 4.2kg. Intramuscular syntometrine has been administered by the midwife. Thirty minutes after delivery of the placenta, she suffers a primary postpartum haemorrhage (PPH) of about 400ml. The most common cause of PPH in this scenario is:

a. An atonic uterus.
b. Coagulopathy.
c. Retained placental tissue.
d. A vaginal tear.
e. A perineal tear.

14 A 29-year-old male is admitted to the emergency department following a road traffic accident. Since admission his GCS has been gradually deteriorating and is now 11. Which of the following would warrant an immediate craniotomy in this patient?

a. Status epilepticus.
b. Unilateral pupillary dilatation.
c. Severe headache with neck rigidity.
d. Cerebrospinal fluid rhinorrhoea.
e. Significant hypotension.

15 A woman in preterm labour requires transfer to a hospital with an available neonatal cot as the baby is at risk. Which of the following drugs would be most suitable for tocolysis in this situation?

a. Ritodrine.
b. Glyceryl trinitrate (GTN).
c. Atosiban.
d. Magnesium sulphate.
e. Salbutamol nebuliser.

16 A 32-year-old male who is a known heroin addict, is on the trauma list for open reduction and internal fixation of a fracture of his humerus. He has been abusing heroin for the last 3 years. He is very anxious about postoperative pain relief and the surgeon is concerned about compartment syndrome in the postoperative period. Which of the following is the best choice for postoperative pain relief?

a. Multimodal analgesia with 'PRN' morphine.
b. Multimodal analgesia with an additional infraclavicular brachial plexus block using 20ml of 0.25% bupivacaine.
c. Multimodal analgesia with a morphine PCA.
d. Multimodal analgesia with an intravenous infusion of morphine.
e. Fentanyl patch with an initial dose of 50µg/hr.

17 A woman without past psychiatric history develops severe postnatal depression and commits suicide 30 days after giving birth. According to the Centre for Maternal and Child Enquiries (formerly CEMACH), this death is best classified as:

a. Late, direct maternal death.
b. Late, indirect maternal death.
c. Indirect maternal death.
d. Direct maternal death.
e. Coincidental maternal death.

18 A 26-year-old male patient is admitted to the intensive care unit following a severe head injury. On admission the baseline blood results show: K^+ 3.4mmol/L, Na^+ 136mmol/L and Cl^- 112mmol/L. He has been intubated, sedated and hyperventilated for the last hour. His arterial blood gas reveals a $PaCO_2$ of 3.3kPa. His ECG morphology on the monitor has now changed with ST segment depression, T-wave flattening and occasional premature ventricular contractions. The most likely cause for the ECG changes is:

a.   Increased intracranial pressure.
b.   Hypokalaemia.
c.   Myocardial ischaemia.
d.   Hyperkalaemia.
e.   Hyponatraemia.

19 You have inserted a central venous catheter via the right internal jugular vein in a 40-year-old male patient about to undergo a laparotomy. The best method to confirm the correct placement of this central venous catheter would be:

a.   Measurement of pH of the blood sample drawn from the catheter.
b.   Measurement of $PaCO_2$.
c.   Measurement of pressure in the catheter using a pressure transducer.
d.   Chest X-ray.
e.   Aspiration of dark red blood from all the lumens of the catheter.

20 A 45-year-old woman complains of gradual increasing numbness and paraesthesia in the thumb, index and middle fingers, more severe at night. Clinical examination reveals wasting of the muscles of the thenar eminence. These clinical features suggest compression of the following structure in the wrist:

a.   Median nerve.
b.   Ulnar nerve.
c.   Superficial radial nerve.

d. Ulnar artery.
e. Radial artery.

21 A 49-year-old male presents with a history of pain along the lower jaw on the left side. The pain is paroxysmal, shooting, and very intense and lasts for a few seconds to minutes. In between the episodes, he has no residual abnormal sensation. The pain is brought on by brushing his teeth, shaving or at times, by touch. In the first instance, what would be the most appropriate action in his medical management?

a. Arrange for an urgent MRI brain scan.
b. Commence treatment with carbamazepine.
c. Refer the patient to a neurosurgeon.
d. Prescribe fentanyl lozenges.
e. Refer the patient to a psychologist.

22 A 72-year-old male patient underwent elective decompression of the lumbar spine. He had no previous experience of general anaesthesia. Tracheal intubation was difficult due to a grade 3 view of the larynx. A gum elastic bougie was successfully placed in the trachea at the third attempt at direct laryngoscopy and a size 8.5mm endotracheal tube was railroaded over the bougie with some difficulty. In the recovery room the patient was noted to have inspiratory stridor with an oxygen saturation of 92%. The oxygen saturation rose to 97% following administration of nebulised adrenaline. Which of the following is the most likely cause of his symptoms?

a. Airway oedema.
b. Vocal cord paralysis.
c. Arytenoid subluxation.
d. Laryngospasm.
e. Arytenoid dislocation.

+ 23 A 64-year-old male was listed for a lumbar laminectomy in the prone position. Following pre-oxygenation, general anaesthesia was induced using propofol and atracurium by a trainee anaesthetist. The trainee anaesthetist encountered a difficult intubation due to a grade 4 view of the larynx and the airway was secured using a laryngeal mask airway (LMA). Help was summoned from a consultant anaesthetist. The most suitable method of performing tracheal intubation by the second anaesthetist would be:

a.   Waking up the patient and performing an awake fibreoptic intubation.

b.   Performing a fibreoptic-assisted intubation through the LMA.

c.   Removing the LMA and attempting direct laryngoscopy.

d.   Removing the LMA, inserting an intubating LMA and attempting tracheal intubation.

e.   Replacing the LMA with a 'Proseal' LMA to facilitate positive pressure ventilation.

- 24 A 68-year-old male patient is admitted to the intensive care unit (ICU) with lethargy and shortness of breath. His past medical history includes hypertension, non-insulin-dependent diabetes, ischaemic heart disease, and impaired renal function. His current medication includes metformin and gliclazide. Soon after admission to the ICU, he is sedated, intubated and ventilated. The subsequent blood gas analysis reveals a pH of 7.08 and a lactate of 18mmol/L. The most appropriate measure to correct the acidosis includes:

a.   Intravenous sodium bicarbonate.

b.   Haemodialysis.

c.   Intravenous insulin.

d.   Hyperventilation.

e.   Tri-hydroxymethyl aminomethane (THAM).

25 A 68-year-old male patient is admitted to the intensive care unit with lethargy and intermittent disorientation. His past medical history includes depression and hypertension. On admission the baseline electrolytes show a low sodium (105mmol/L) and low potassium

(3.1mmol/L). During the first 24 hours, 3L of 0.9% sodium chloride with 20mmol/L of potassium chloride are administered, and subsequently, enteral nutrition is started. Five days later the patient becomes increasingly drowsy despite a normal serum sodium level. Which of the following investigations would be most useful in establishing the diagnosis?

a. Serum potassium level.
b. CSF proteins.
c. Electroencephalogram.
d. Magnetic resonance imaging of the brain.
e. Brain stem evoked potentials.

11

26 A 67-year-old patient has had a total knee replacement. He is on morphine PCA for the management of postoperative pain. He has received a total of 40mg morphine in the recovery area and you are worried that he may develop an opioid overdose. Which of the following is the earliest sign of opioid overdose?

a. Respiratory rate less than 8 per minute.
b. A fall in oxygen saturation.
c. Rapid shallow breathing.
d. Progressive rise in sedation level.
e. Uncontrolled vomiting.

27 A 35-year-old male patient has been admitted to ITU with Guillain Barré syndrome. You have inserted a fine-bore nasogastric (NG) tube for enteral feeding. Prior to commencing feeding, which of the following is the best test to confirm the correct placement of a nasogastric tube?

a. Injection of 50ml of air with auscultation over the stomach ('whoosh' test).
b. Chest X-ray.
c. Aspiration of at least 10ml through the NG tube.
d. Checking the pH of the aspirate.
e. Abdominal X-ray.

28 A 30-year-old, obese, primiparous woman has requested epidural analgesia for labour pain. After obtaining consent the epidural space was located at a depth of 7cm with loss of resistance to saline. A catheter was inserted successfully into the epidural space through a Tuohy needle despite initial slight resistance. On removal of the needle it was noted that the catheter had broken at the 6cm mark and the missing segment was not seen either on the drapes or on the floor. The most important step in the further management of the broken epidural catheter is:

a.   CT scan of the lumbar region.
b.   Plain X-ray of the lumbar region.
c.   Neurosurgical referral.
d.   Surgical exploration of the back for the missing segment of catheter.
e.   Perform an epidural at a different space.

29 A 12-year-old girl is undergoing scoliosis correction. Anaesthesia is maintained with isoflurane in nitrous oxide and oxygen. A total of 10mg morphine has been administered as intermittent boluses. About 30 minutes into the procedure, the patient develops a tachycardia which is not responsive to a bolus of intravenous fluids or intravenous morphine. The $EtCO_2$ is 7.2kPa despite adequate ventilation and the temperature is recorded as 39°C. The first step in the immediate treatment should be:

a.   Dantrolene sodium 1mg/kg as an initial bolus.
b.   Dantrolene sodium 2-3mg/kg as an initial bolus.
c.   Send urine sample for myoglobin.
d.   Measurement of arterial blood pH.
e.   Insertion of central venous line.

30 A 65-year-old male patient is undergoing laser excision of a laryngeal papilloma. The airway is secured with a 'Laser-flex' endotracheal tube. During the procedure the proximal cuff is burst by a laser beam

and a small flame of fire appears in the surgical field. The most appropriate immediate measure should be:

a. Increasing the inspired oxygen concentration.
b. Continuing with laser resection to complete the procedure as soon as possible.
c. Flooding the field with normal saline.
d. Increasing the nitrous oxide concentration in order to reduce the inspired oxygen concentration.
e. Changing the endotracheal tube immediately.

Set 1 answers

1 Answer: D. Intubate and ventilate the patient with 100% oxygen.

The history and examination findings indicate that the most likely cause of unconsciousness in this patient is carbon monoxide (CO) poisoning. Carboxy-haemoglobin (COHb) has a similar absorption spectrum to oxyhaemoglobin and therefore oxygen saturation is falsely raised. Carbon monoxide binds with haemoglobin about 250 times as avidly as oxygen and this adversely affects the oxygen content of blood. The half-life of COHb is 4 hours; it is reduced to an hour with 100% oxygen and to 20-30 minutes with hyperbaric oxygen therapy. This patient is unconscious which indicates severe CO poisoning. Airway protection and oxygenation of tissue is an absolute priority and this will be best achieved by tracheal intubation and ventilation with 100% oxygen.

Further reading
1. Piantadosi CA. Carbon monoxide poisoning. *Undersea Hyperb Med* 2004; 31: 167-77.

2 Answer: D. Synchronised DC shock.

Atrial fibrillation (AF) is a commonly encountered arrhythmia postoperatively following cardiothoracic surgery. Lack of co-ordinated atrial contraction results in impulses from different parts of the atria reaching the AV node in rapid succession and only some of these are transmitted. A fast ventricular rate results in inadequate ventricular filling and reduced cardiac output. The management of AF depends on its duration, any obvious correctable causes, evidence of haemodynamic compromise and the coagulation status. Acute onset AF with haemodynamic compromise is best treated by synchronised DC shock to restore sinus rhythm. If the patient's blood pressure is not affected, correctable causes should be addressed, and amiodarone boluses given (5mg/kg over 30 minutes), followed by an infusion (15mg/kg over 23 hours). Anticoagulation should be considered if AF has persisted for more than 2-3 days, especially prior to cardioversion.

Further reading

1. Bajpai A, Rowland E. Atrial fibrillation. *British Journal of Anaesthesia CEACCP* 2006; 6: 219-24.

3   Answer: D. von Willebrand's disease.

von Willebrand's disease is the most commonly inherited (autosomal dominant) coagulation disorder. von Willebrand Factor is a protein involved in platelet adhesion and transfer of coagulation of Factor VIII. Abnormality of this factor leads to abnormal platelet adhesiveness leading to epistaxis, bruising and haemarthrosis. The coagulation profile reveals a prolonged bleeding time and APTT with normal PT and platelet count. Antiplatelet drugs should be avoided and peri-operative use of fresh frozen plasma, cryoprecipitate and desmopressin (which increases Factor VIII and von Willebrand Factor) may be required.

Further reading

1. Geil JD. von Willebrand disease. (http://emedicine.medscape.com/article/959825-overview).

2. von Willebrand's disease. In: *Anaesthesia and intensive care A-Z. An encyclopaedia of principles and practice*, 4th ed, Yentis SM, Hirsch NP, Smith GB, Eds. Oxford, UK: Butterworth-Heinemann, 2009; 600.

4   Answer: C. Serum lipase.

Serum amylase is a non-specific test and is elevated in bowel perforation, obstruction and ischaemia, diabetic ketoacidosis, and pneumonia or neoplasms. Serum lipase levels are more sensitive and specific than amylase in acute pancreatitis and are elevated for up to 14 days. Urinary trypsinogen-2 'Dipstix' testing is still being studied as a test for both confirmation of diagnosis and as an indicator of severity.

Further reading
1. Young SP, Thompson JP. Severe acute pancreatitis. *British Journal of Anaesthesia CEACCP* 2008; 8: 125-8.

5   Answer: B. Spinal anaesthesia.

Complete spinal cord transection leads to loss of all sensation below the level of injury. These patients still, however, have very active local spinal reflexes and this can lead to autonomic hyper-reflexia. The stimuli for autonomic hyper-reflexia are usually perineal procedures such as urinary catheterization. Autonomic hyper-reflexia may present as a severe tachyarrhythmia and hypertension. Autonomic hyper-reflexia can be best avoided by administration of spinal anaesthesia. Postoperative pain after haemorrhoidectomy should not be a significant problem in this patient as the surgery is below the T10 level.

Further reading
1. Teasdale A. Neuromuscular disorders. In: *Oxford handbook of anaesthesia*, 1st ed. Allman KG, Wilson IH, Eds. Oxford, UK: Oxford University Press, 2003; Chapter 9: 180-5.

6   Answer: E. Post-herpetic neuralgia.

Post-herpetic neuralgia (PHN) is pain occurring after *Herpes zoster* infection. After the initial infection, the virus remains dormant in the ganglion of the affected nerve. Reactivation of the virus occurs due to immunosuppression and therefore is more commonly seen in the elderly, and in patients with poor nutrition, malignancy, and immunosuppression due to any cause. The onset of pain is typically followed by the skin rash in the distribution of the affected nerve. The ophthalmic division of the trigeminal nerve is the second most commonly affected nerve; the thoracic dermatome being the commonest. PHN pain is neuropathic in nature and can be treated by using 5% lidocaine plasters, tricyclic antidepressant medication (amitriptyline), calcium channel blockers (gabapentin, pregabalin), sodium channel blockers (phenytoin, carbamazepine) and non-pharmacological therapies such as TENS, acupuncture and cognitive behavioural therapy (CBT).

Further reading
1. Dainty P. Prevention and medical management of post-herpetic neuralgia. *British Journal of Hospital Medicine* 2008; 69: 275-8.

7   Answer: C. Etomidate.

Taking into consideration the history of this patient it would be most appropriate to use etomidate, which is an intravenous anaesthetic agent with the lowest incidence of allergic reactions. The incidence of hypersensitivity reactions amongst induction agents is shown in Table 1.

Table 1. The incidence of hypersensitivity reactions amongst induction agents.

IV anaesthetic agent	Incidence
Propofol	1: 80,000
Thiopentone	1: 20,000 to 40,000
Etomidate	1: 450,000
Ketamine	1: 150,000
Methohexitone	1: 7,000 to 15,000

Further reading
1. Aitkenhead AR. Intravenous anaesthetic agents. In: *Textbook of anaesthesia*, 5th ed. Aitkenhead AR, Rowbothom DJ, Smith G, Eds. London, UK: Churchill Livingstone, 2007; Chapter 3: 34-51.

8   Answer: D. Air embolism.

Air embolism is a well recognised complication of surgery during any operation in which the operative site is higher than the right atrium. Venous air embolism (VAE) causes pulmonary microvascular occlusion resulting in increased physiological dead space. Bronchoconstriction may also develop. Other signs include hypotension, arrhythmia, increased pulmonary artery pressure and decreased $EtCO_2$. VAE can be diagnosed by detection of a sudden reduction in $EtCO_2$, a decrease in blood pressure, and use of a Doppler, precordial stethoscope (millwheel murmur), or a transoesophageal stethoscope. Treatment is supportive and includes informing the surgeon to flood the operative field with saline, discontinuation of nitrous oxide if in use and increasing the FiO_2 to 1.0. To increase the venous pressure, PEEP should be applied and if possible the position of the operative site should be changed to a level below the heart. Blood pressure should be supported using intravenous fluids and vasopressors. If a large volume of air has entered the circulation and the surgical condition permits, the patient should be turned into the left lateral position in an attempt to keep the air in the right atrium and aspiration performed via a central line if present.

Further reading

1. Clayton T, Manara A. Neurosurgery. In: *Oxford handbook of anaesthesia*, 1st ed. Allman KG, Wilson IH, Eds. Oxford, UK: Oxford University Press, 2003; Chapter 19: 418-9.

9   Answer: A. Analysis of blood or stool for botulinum toxin.

The history is suggestive of botulism. The best diagnostic test is to identify the toxin in blood or stools. Other conditions which may present similarly include:

- Poliomyelitis: a febrile illness with asymmetric paralysis. Diagnosis is by virus culture.
- Guillain Barré syndrome: a febrile illness with loss of sensation. Diagnosis is by CSF analysis and electrophysiological studies.

19

♦ Myasthenia gravis: a fluctuating weakness, which is diagnosed by the 'Tensilon' test.

Further reading
1. Wenham T, Cohen A. Botulism. *British Journal of Anaesthesia CEACCP* 2008; 8: 21-5.

10 Answer: D. Stop enoxaparin and start an alternative anticoagulant.

This patient's history is suggestive of heparin-induced thrombocytopaenia (HIT). HIT is an adverse drug reaction to heparin. Adverse reactions are either non-immune-mediated (type I) or immune-mediated (type II). The non-immune mediated reaction typically has an earlier onset and seldom leads to a drop in the platelet count below 100 x 10^9/L. The immune-mediated reaction is clinically more significant as it is associated with thrombosis. It occurs between 5-14 days post-heparin exposure and this is known as 'typical' HIT. The incidence of HIT is estimated at 1% with low-molecular-weight heparins (LMWH) and about 5% with unfractionated heparins (UFH). HIT has been described with every route of heparin administration. Diagnosis of HIT requires a low threshold of suspicion. Other features include a systemic response to heparin injection and overt disseminated intravascular coagulopathy. Where clinical suspicion of HIT is intermediate to high, it is essential to stop UFH or LMWH. There should be no delay in commencing anticoagulation with alternative agents while awaiting confirmatory tests, as the risk of thrombosis remains as high as 50% even after stopping heparin.

Further reading
1. Warkentin TE. Heparin-induced thrombocytopaenia: diagnosis and management. *Circulation* 2004; 110: 454-8.

11 Answer: C. Intrathecal saddle neurolytic block.

Cancer pain can be successfully managed in about 90% of patients using the WHO analgesic ladder. In the remaining 10% of patients, interventional therapy may be required. The nature of pain can be both nociceptive and neuropathic. At times, the tolerance to opioid medication leads to poor pain control and 'opioid rotation' may be effective in such cases. In this patient switching MST to equivalent doses of oxycodone ('opioid rotation') and increasing the opioid medication dose has been already tried but without satisfactory response. The next appropriate step would be an interventional therapy. Coeliac plexus block is effective only for abdominal malignancy and is therefore not a suitable option. Lumbar sympathectomy is generally effective for lower limb pain. In this particular patient, intrathecal neurolysis, using hyperbaric phenol to provide a saddle block, would be most appropriate. It can cause leg numbness but this can be avoided by carefully restricting it to a saddle block. Alcohol is hypobaric compared to CSF and can also be used for neurolysis in the management of malignant pain.

Further reading

1. Medicis E, Laon-Casasoal OA. Neurolytic blocks. *Clinical pain management - practical applications and procedures*, 1st ed. Breivik H, Campbell W, Eccleston C, Eds. London, UK: Arnold, 2002; Chapter 19: 247-54.

12 Answer: B. Intravenous magnesium sulphate infusion, following a loading dose.

This woman has severe pre-eclampsia, as defined by the level of both systolic and diastolic hypertension and presence of cerebral symptoms. She is at risk of eclampsia. The MAGPIE study has demonstrated that administration of magnesium sulphate (loading dose over 1 hour followed by infusion) to women with pre-eclampsia reduces the risk of an eclamptic seizure by over 50%. It should be continued for 24 hours following delivery or 24 hours after the last seizure, whichever is the later. Sublingual nifedipine is not recommended. Other antihypertensive agents to consider are oral nifedipine, an intravenous labetalol infusion and intravenous hydralazine. In this case, epidural analgesia is not required as the woman is not in labour and a Caesarean section is planned.

Further reading

1. RCOG Green-Top 10A guideline: The management of severe pre-eclampsia/eclampsia. (www.rcog.org.uk).

21

2. Magpie Trial Collaborative Group: Do women with pre-eclampsia, and their babies, benefit from magnesium sulphate? The Magpie Trial: a randomised placebo-controlled trial. *Lancet* 2002; 359: 1877-90.

13 Answer: A. An atonic uterus.

The most common cause of primary (within 24 hours) postpartum haemorrhage is an atonic uterus, occurring in about 70% of cases. The other options mentioned above are possible causes which need to be excluded. In particular, tears may cause significant haemorrhage and can be more difficult to diagnose if high in the genital tract, often requiring an examination under anaesthesia. Factors predisposing to an atonic uterus include a large baby (in this case), multiple pregnancy, prolonged labour (especially if augmented with syntocinon), abnormal placentation, multiparity, and chorioamnionitis.

14 Answer: B. Unilateral pupillary dilatation.

Traumatic head injury is considered to be severe if the GCS is gradually deteriorating. The usual clinical presentation of an extradural haematoma is severe headache, loss of consciousness with or without a lucid interval and rapid development of a fixed dilated pupil on the side of the injury with contralateral hemiparesis. Extradural haematoma occurs due to rupture of the middle meningeal artery. It occurs in approximately 10% of severe head injuries. Immediate surgery is required to evacuate the haematoma. Severe head injury can lead to status epilepticus and it may indicate the need for intubation and ventilation, but not surgery. CSF rhinorrhoea is associated with a base of skull fracture and surgery may be required if it does not stop spontaneously.

Further reading

1. Lannoo E, Van Rietvelde F, Colardyn F, *et al*. Early predictors of mortality and morbidity after severe closed head injury. *J Neurotrauma* 2000; 17: 403-14.
2. Triage, assessment, investigation and early management of head injury in infants, children and adults. NICE guidelines CG 56, September 2007. (http://www.nice.org.uk/CG56).

15 Answer: C. Atosiban.

Preterm birth is defined as that occurring before 37 completed weeks, but most mortality and morbidity is experienced in babies born before 34 weeks. Ritodrine has predominantly β2-receptor effects, relaxing the muscles in the uterus, arterioles and bronchi. It is not recommended as it is associated with a relatively high incidence of pulmonary oedema. Atosiban (an oxytocin receptor antagonist) and nifedipine appear to have comparable effectiveness in delaying delivery for a few days, with fewer maternal adverse effects and less risk of rare serious adverse events. Nifedipine has the advantage of oral use and it is cheap. However, it is not licensed in the UK for use as a tocolytic. Though both magnesium sulphate and GTN have a relaxant effect on the uterus, their use in this situation is not recommended as frequent monitoring of blood pressure and other vital parameters will be required. A salbutamol nebuliser will only have a transient effect on the uterus.

Further reading
1. RCOG Green-Top 1B guideline: Tocolytic drugs for women in preterm labour. (www.rcog.org.uk).

16 Answer: C. Multimodal analgesia with a morphine PCA.

Acute postoperative pain relief is a challenging issue in patients on long-term opioids or with opioid addiction. In these patients, non-opioid analgesics should be used if possible and if opioid analgesics are indicated, then fast onset, short-acting opioids are preferred to allow dose adjustment. Partial agonist (e.g. buprenorphine) and agonist-antagonist (e.g. pentazocine) opioid drugs should be avoided. The use of a morphine PCA allows dose titration in a safer way and also helps to avoid possible patient confrontation with health care professionals. In patients with unmanageable pain after high doses of morphine, a ketamine infusion can be used in a dose of 0.2 to 0.3mg/kg/hr for 24 to 48 hours and it may, by its NMDA antagonist action, reverse opioid tolerance in addition to its analgesic action. Regional analgesia using a brachial plexus block may mask the clinical signs of compartment syndrome.

Further reading
1. Mehta V, Langford RM. Acute pain management for opioid-dependent patients. *Anaesthesia* 2006; 61: 269-76.

17 Answer: C. Indirect maternal death.

This is a maternal death occurring within 42 days of the end of pregnancy. The suicide was related to the pregnancy, but there is no obstetric cause and so the death is classified as an indirect maternal death. In the last two triennial reports, suicide has been the leading cause of maternal death overall.

Table 2. Definition of maternal deaths.	
Maternal deaths	Deaths of women while pregnant or within 42 days of the end of the pregnancy, from any cause related to or aggravated by the pregnancy or its management, but not from accidental or incidental causes
Direct	Deaths resulting from obstetric complications of the pregnant state (pregnancy, labour and puerperium), from interventions, omissions, incorrect treatment or from a chain of events resulting from any of the above
Indirect	Deaths resulting from previous existing disease, or disease that developed during pregnancy and which was not due to direct obstetric causes, but which was aggravated by the physiologic effects of pregnancy
Late	Deaths occurring between 42 days and 1 year after abortion, miscarriage or delivery that are due to direct or indirect maternal causes
Coincidental (fortuitous)	Deaths from unrelated causes which happen to occur in pregnancy or the puerperium

Further reading

1. Why mothers die 2000-2002; http://www.cmace.org.uk/Publications/ Saving-Mothers-Lives-Report-2000-2002.aspx.

18 Answer: B. Hypokalaemia.

Hypokalaemia is the most likely cause for the ECG abnormality because:

♦ The baseline plasma potassium level is low at only 3.4mmol/L.
♦ Hyperventilation leading to respiratory alkalosis can shift the potassium into the cells, thereby reducing the potassium in the extracellular fluid and further lowering the plasma potassium.
♦ The ECG abnormalities of hypokalaemia include T-wave inversion, ST segment depression, a prolonged PR interval and prominent U waves.

25

Further reading

1. Hypokalaemia. In: *ECG diagnosis made easy.* Vecht RJ, Ed. Martin Dunitz, 2001: 185.
2. Abnormal potassium balance. In: *Lecture notes on fluid and electrolyte balance*, 2nd ed. Willatts SM, Ed. Oxford, UK: Blackwell Scientific Publications, 1987; Chapter 8: 167-76.

19 Answer: D. Chest X-ray.

A chest X-ray should confirm the correct placement of a central venous line. The catheter tip should be just above the pericardial reflection, outside the cardiac silhouette. The catheter should be within the superior vena cava (SVC), relatively parallel to the walls of the SVC. The catheter tip should abut against the wall of the SVC. All other mentioned methods in the placement of the catheter may be within the SVC or a major vein.

20 Answer: A. Median nerve.

The clinical features described are suggestive of carpal tunnel syndrome, caused by compression of the median nerve within the carpal tunnel. Initially symptoms appear typically during the night because flexing of the wrist during sleep causes further compression of the median nerve. The contents of the carpal tunnel include the median nerve, the tendon of flexor pollicis longus, and tendons of flexor digitorum superficialis and profundus.

Further reading
1. Nerve and muscle. In: *Lecture notes on neurology,* 7th ed. Ginsberg L, Ed. Oxford, UK: Blackwell Science, 1999; Chapter 17: 146-7.

21 Answer: B. Commence treatment with carbamazepine.

This patient has a classical history of trigeminal neuralgia pain. Trigeminal neuralgia usually presents in middle-aged patients with unilateral neuropathic pain in the distribution of one or more divisions of the trigeminal nerve. Commonly, the maxillary and/or mandibular divisions are affected. The pain lasts for a short period and in between the episodes, there are no symptoms or signs. The pain can be severe enough to induce suicidal thoughts. The exact pathophysiology is not known but in some patients vascular compression of the trigeminal ganglion has been implicated. The pain responds to medications used to treat neuropathic pain in about 70% of patients and traditionally the first-line drug used is carbamazepine. About 15-30% may respond to microvascular decompression of the trigeminal ganglion and this is indicated if the MRI scan shows vascular compression of the ganglion. If the patient does not respond to medication therapy, MRI of the brain can be performed to rule out other pathology.

Further reading
1. Sindrup SH, Jensen TS. Pharmacotherapy of trigeminal neuralgia. *The Clinical Journal of Pain* 2002; 18: 22-7.

22 Answer: A. Airway oedema.

Airway oedema as a result of repeated laryngoscopy and intubation attempts can result in inspiratory stridor along with desaturation. Other differential diagnoses include laryngospasm, arytenoid subluxation or dislocation, but these are unlikely to improve with nebulised adrenaline. A flexible nasendoscopy should confirm the diagnosis. Arytenoid subluxation can be treated with voice therapy.

Further reading
1. Tan V, Seevanayagam S. Arytenoid subluxation after a difficult intubation treated successfully with voice therapy. *Anesthesia and Intensive Care* 2009; 37: 843-6.

23 Answer: B. Performing a fibreoptic-assisted intubation through the LMA.

The 'plan B' of the Difficult Airway Society guidelines includes tracheal intubation through an LMA or intubating LMA. In this case, as the airway is secured and the patient is well oxygenated using the LMA, the most appropriate decision is to perform fibreoptic-assisted tracheal intubation through the LMA. Blind tracheal intubation through an LMA has a low success rate and can cause airway trauma. One-stage fibreoptic intubation performed by directly loading the endotracheal tube over the fibreoptic scope has certain limitations. It requires a longer tube such as a microlaryngoscopy tube or a north facing polar nasal tube. It also limits the size of the endotracheal tube, as the LMA tube only allows an endotracheal tube of up to 6 to 7mm internal diameter depending on the size and type of LMA. A two-stage technique using an Aintree intubation catheter overcomes these limitations. Using an LMA in the prone position would place the patient's airway at risk.

Further reading
1. Henderson JJ, *et al.* Difficult Airway Society guidelines for the management of the unanticipated difficult intubation. *Anaesthesia* 2004; 59: 675-94.

24 Answer: B. Haemodialysis.

This patient has severe lactic acidosis with pre-existing impaired renal function. Metformin is a biguanide oral hypoglycaemic agent. The mechanism of its action involves reduced intestinal absorption of glucose, reduced gluconeogenesis and increased peripheral utilisation of glucose due to increased insulin sensitivity. Biguanides cause type B lactic acidosis by increasing lactic acid production whilst impairing its removal by the kidneys and liver. Metformin is contraindicated in the presence of severe hepatic or renal impairment. Treatment with sodium bicarbonate alone fails to correct acidosis, and may cause intracellular acidosis and hypernatraemia. Haemodialysis or continuous venovenous haemofiltration has been shown to have a better outcome, removing the metformin and correcting the acidosis. Tri-hydroxymethyl aminomethane (THAM) is an organic amine proton acceptor, and should be used with caution in the presence of renal impairment as it is associated with hyperkalaemia.

Further reading

1. Pan LTT, MacLaren G. Continuous venovenous haemofiltration for metformin induced lactic acidosis. *Anesthesia and Intensive Care* 2009; 37: 830-2.
2. Teale KFH, Devine A, *et al.* The managemnet of metformin overdose. *Anaesthesia* 1998; 53: 698-701.

25 Answer: D. Magnetic resonance imaging of the brain.

The most likely cause for the deterioration of this patient is central pontine myelinolysis (CPM). Acute hyponatraemia results in cerebral oedema, due to the inability of neuronal cells to extrude potassium. In chronic hyponatraemia, however, neuronal cells may adapt by extrusion of organic osmolytes from their cytoplasm. Osmotic demyelination is a recognised complication of rapid correction of hyponatraemia. Patients with severe malnutrition, alcoholism, and advanced liver disease are more susceptible to CPM. In order to avoid CPM, it is recommended that during the first 24 hours the total increase in serum sodium should not exceed 20mmol/L. The diagnosis can be confirmed by an MRI scan (T2 weighed images), which would show high intensity lesions (bright areas) in the region of the central pons. Normally there is symmetric, non-inflammatory demyelination in the central part of the pons. In 10% of patients with central pontine myelinolysis, however, demyelination also occurs in extrapontine regions, including the midbrain, thalamus, basal nuclei and cerebellum.

Further reading

1. Luzzio C. Central pontine myelinosis: differential diagnosis and workup. (http://emedicine.medscape.com/article/1174329-overview).

2. Schuster M, Diekmann S, *et al*. Central pontine myelinosis despite slow sodium rise in a case of severe community-acquired hyponatraemia. *Anesthesia and Intensive Care* 2009; 37: 117-20.

26 Answer: D. Progressive rise in sedation level.

Opioids are commonly used in the management of intra-operative and postoperative pain. Excessive doses of opioid initially cause rising sedation levels, confusion, nightmares, hallucinations and at this stage delaying a further dose or reducing the dose is enough to alleviate the problem. If not recognized, the patient will develop respiratory depression followed by a decrease in oxygen saturation. Oxygen saturation changes may not be evident in the early stages especially if the patient is on supplementary oxygen.

29

Further reading

1. Tran ML, Warfield C. Opioid analgesics. In: *Clinical pain management - practical applications and procedures*, 1st ed. Breivik H, Campbell W, Eccleston C, Eds. London, UK: Arnold, 2002; Chapter 6: 59-76.

27 Answer: B. Chest X-ray.

It is essential to ensure the correct position of the NG tube prior to commencing feeding through it. A chest X-ray is the best method to confirm the correct placement. Although the other mentioned methods may indicate the placement of the tube in the stomach, they are not always reliable. It may be difficult to hear the 'whoosh' sound on injecting air in obese patients.

Further reading

1. Reducing the harm caused by nasogastric tubes - interim advice for health care staff, 2005. (http://www.baxa.com/resources/docs/research /NPSAConfPosofNG.pdf).

28 Answer: A. CT scan of the lumbar region.

The epidural catheter is radio-opaque; it may be visible on plain X-ray but a CT scan is the most helpful in delineating the location of the broken catheter tip. The catheter fragment is unlikely to cause any further problems to the patient, but fibrosis around the nerve root may produce signs of radicular irritation. An immediate management plan for labour analgesia should be instituted. This may include discussion with the patient and obstetrician and depends on the progress of labour. Alternate modes of analgesia and performing another epidural should be considered.

Further reading
1. Fragneto RY. The broken epidural catheter: an anesthesiologist's dilemma. *Journal of Clinical Anesthesia* 2007; 19: 243-4.

29 Answer: B. Dantrolene sodium 2-3mg/kg as an initial bolus.

The clinical scenario is suggestive of malignant hyperthermia (MH): unexplained tachycardia, an increase in $EtCO_2$ and hyperthermia. The correct dose of dantrolene is 2-3mg/kg as an initial bolus followed by 1mg/kg PRN. The other immediate measures include removing the trigger agent, and maintaining anaesthesia with total intravenous anaesthesia. Active cooling measures and intravenous infusion of cold I.V. fluids should be performed. End-tidal CO_2, invasive arterial BP, CVP, core and peripheral temperature, urine output and pH, arterial blood gases, potassium, haematocrit, platelets, clotting indices, and creatine kinase should be monitored. The systemic effects of MH include hyperkalaemia, cardiac arrhythmias, myoglobinaemia and disseminated intravascular coagulation.

Further reading
1. Guidelines for the management of malignant hyperthermia crisis. The Association of Anaesthetists of Great Britain and Ireland, 2007.

30 Answer: C. Flooding the field with normal saline.

The main components of the 'fire triangle' include fuel, oxygen and energy. The 'Laser flex' endotracheal tube is a metallic tube with two cuffs. Both cuffs need to be filled with saline. The cuff part of the tube can act as a fuel. The laser beam acts as a source of energy. Both oxygen and nitrous oxide supports combustion. The mixture of oxygen and nitrous oxide is more flammable than an oxygen and air mixture. A lowest possible inspired oxygen concentration should be used during laser surgery of the airway.

1. Kitching AJ, Edge CJ. Lasers and surgery. *British Journal of Anaesthesia CPD review* 2003; 8: 143-6.

Set 2 questions

1   A 50-year-old female patient with a history of non-insulin-dependent diabetes has undergone trans-sphenoidal excision of a pituitary adenoma. During the immediate postoperative period she develops polyuria with a urine output of 600ml over 2 hours. The urine osmolarity is 320mosmol/L and the specific gravity is 1.001. The most appropriate treatment for this patient is:

a.   Intravenous 0.9% sodium chloride.
b.   Intravenous DDAVP.
c.   Intravenous glucose.
d.   Intravenous insulin.
e.   Intravenous glucose and potassium.

2   A 48-year-old female patient involved in a road traffic accident about 36 hours ago is scheduled for an open reduction of bilateral mandibular fractures. She complains of neck pain and cervical spine injury is suspected. The best possible investigation to exclude cervical spine injury is:

a.   Cervical spine X-ray lateral view.
b.   Cervical spine X-ray anteroposterior view.
c.   MRI scan of the cervical spine.
d.   Helical CT with sagittal reformat.
e.   Dynamic fluoroscopy.

3   A 53-year-old female patient is anaesthetised for an emergency laparotomy. She is obese with a BMI of 39. After induction of anaesthesia a central venous catheter is placed via the right subclavian vein following two failed attempts via the right internal jugular vein. About 30 minutes after starting the procedure, the airway pressure and heart rate increase and the oxygen saturation decreases to 88%. The most likely cause is:

a.   A displaced endotracheal tube.
b.   Severe bronchospasm.
c.   Kinking of the endotracheal tube.
d.   Anaphylaxis.
e.   Tension pneumothorax.

4   A 69-year-old male patient is admitted to the intensive care unit following emergency repair of a leaking abdominal aortic aneurysm. On admission to the unit, he is hypotensive, and requires inotropic support. The urine output over the last 12 hours is only 30mL. Blood and urine analysis reveal: creatinine – 545mmol/L, urine osmolality – 165mmol/L and a urine: plasma creatinine ratio of 25. The most likely cause of the low urine output is:

a.   Intrinsic renal failure.
b.   Severe dehydration.
c.   Pre-renal type of renal failure.
d.   Post-renal type of failure.
e.   Adrenal failure with hypotension.

5   A 50-year-old male patient has been admitted to the high dependency unit following surgery for bilateral fractures of the lower limbs. His medical history includes bipolar disorder and mild hypertension, and he is treated with lithium 400mg per day and bendrofluazide 2.5mg per day. During the intra-operative period, gentamicin 240mg and flucloxacillin 1g is administered as antibiotic prophylaxis. Since admission to the unit he has developed significant polyuria with a urine output of 200-400ml per hour for the past 6

hours. There is no myoglobin in the urine. The most likely cause for his polyuria is:

a.   Rhabdomyolysis.
b.   Central diabetes insipidus.
c.   Nephrogenic diabetes insipidus.
d.   Bendrofluazide.
e.   Antibiotic therapy.

6   You have been asked to review a 67-year-old patient on the fourth postoperative day, who is complaining of severe back pain and increasing numbness in both legs developing over the previous few hours. He has had an epidural *in situ* since his operation; the epidural infusion was switched off 8 hours ago as his blood pressure had been low. For the last few hours his temperature has been 38°C. Your first step in the management of this patient should be:

a.   Give an epidural top-up using 0.5% bupivacaine.
b.   Remove the epidural catheter and start morphine PCA.
c.   Arrange for an MRI scan of the spine.
d.   Arrange for surgical review as soon as possible.
e.   Start multimodal analgesia and broad spectrum antibiotics.

7   A 75-year-old male patient had a transurethral resection of the prostate under spinal anaesthesia 2 weeks ago. He now presents with weakness of the left foot. On clinical examination he has loss of sensation over the dorsum of the left foot and motor power is grade 3/5 for dorsiflexion of the left foot. The most useful investigation in establishing the diagnosis would be:

a.   MRI scan of the lumbar spine.
b.   Fasting blood glucose.
c.   A complete neurological examination.
d.   CT scan of the lumbar spine.
e.   Electromyography.

8 A 65-year-old female patient with a history of ischaemic heart disease is scheduled for a laparoscopic cholecystectomy. A 12-lead ECG has been performed as part of a routine pre-operative assessment. Which of the following abnormal findings is most likely to be present on the ECG?

a. Tall R waves in leads V5 and V6.
b. ST-T wave abnormalities.
c. Pathological Q waves.
d. Right bundle branch block.
e. Deep S waves in lead V1.

9 A 45-year-old man presents to the emergency department with severe constant epigastric pain radiating to the back and flanks, and vomiting. Examination reveals pyrexia, abdominal distension, rebound tenderness and discolouration of the flanks. Blood tests reveal elevated lipase and amylase levels. Which one of the following is the recommended investigation for an initial assessment?

a. Biliary tract ultrasound.
b. X-ray abdomen.
c. Angiography.
d. CT scan.
e. MRI scan.

10 A 30-year-old male is undergoing a laparotomy for a ruptured spleen, liver laceration and bowel injury following a road traffic accident. The estimated blood loss so far is 4L. During the procedure 8 units of packed red cells and 3L of Hartmann's solution have been infused. There is increased bleeding from the wound edge and from the site of venous access. The following laboratory test supports the diagnosis of DIC rather than dilutional coagulopathy:

a. Haemoglobin.
b. D-Dimer.
c. Platelet count.
d. Bleeding time.
e. INR.

11 A 48-year-old male lorry driver presents with severe right-sided sciatica which he has suffered from for the last 9 months. He has already tried treatment with analgesics, physiotherapy and acupuncture. His MRI scan shows moderate disc prolapse at the L5-S1 level. He does not wish to undergo any surgical intervention. The most suitable treatment is:

a. Stronger opioid medication.
b. Facet joint injection.
c. Epidural steroid injection.
d. Traction therapy to the lumbar spine.
e. Six weeks' bed rest.

12 A 50-year-old female patient has had a parathyroidectomy for hyperparathyroidism secondary to chronic renal failure. She has a history of arthritis, backache and neck pain. In the recovery room, she complains of weakness in all four limbs. The clinical examination reveals reduced power in all four limbs and reduced sensation below the C6 dermatome. The most useful investigation in establishing the cause of weakness would be:

a. CT scan of the head.
b. MRI scan of the cervical spine.
c. Serum calcium level.
d. MRI scan of the head.
e. Electromyography.

13 A 4-week baby with a history of projectile vomiting for the last few days has been diagnosed with pyloric stenosis. Which one of the following parameters is most likely to suggest severe volume depletion?

a. Urine output of 0.5ml/hour.
b. Serum sodium 129mmol/L.
c. Metabolic alkalosis with alkaline urine.
d. Metabolic alkalosis with acidic urine.
e. Serum chloride 100mmol/L.

14 A 60-year-old male patient with a history of hypertension and ischaemic heart disease is scheduled for a carotid endarterectomy under general anaesthesia. Which of the following would be the most appropriate monitor of peri-operative cerebral ischaemia?

a. Electro-encephalography.
b. Somatosensory evoked potentials.
c. Transcranial Doppler.
d. Motor evoked potentials.
e. Auditory evoked potentials.

15 A 68-year-old male with known hypertension and a long-term smoker has been diagnosed with bronchogenic carcinoma and is being assessed for his suitability for a right-sided pneumonectomy. His post-bronchodilator FEV1 is 1.6L. Which one of the following tests should be performed next to assess suitability for the pneumonectomy?

a. Best distance on two shuttle walk test.
b. Arterial blood gas analysis.
c. Cardiopulmonary exercise test.
d. Pulmonary function tests to estimate postoperative FEV1.
e. CT scan of the chest.

16 A 7-year-old boy is in severe pain and distress in the recovery room following urgent open reduction and internal fixation of a fractured radius. He is awake and is tachycardic. Intra-operative analgesia included fentanyl 3µg/kg I.V., paracetamol 500mg rectally and diclofenac 25mg rectally. What would be the most appropriate analgesic option for him now?

a. Intravenous morphine infusion at 10µg/kg/hour.
b. Intramuscular codeine phosphate 1mg/kg.
c. Axillary brachial plexus block.
d. Morphine 100µg/kg as an intravenous bolus.
e. Administer entonox until he calms down.

17 A 57-year-old female is due to undergo urgent surgery for internal fixation of a fractured humerus. She is known to have primary hyperparathyroidism. Pre-operative blood results and the ECG are unremarkable except for a serum calcium level of 3.3mmol/L. Which initial therapy should be used to treat hypercalcaemia in this patient?

a. Intravenous corticosteroids.
b. Intravenous saline and furosemide.
c. Intravenous calcitonin.
d. Haemodialysis.
e. Intravenous biphosphonates.

18 A 53-year-old female patient is undergoing a total hip replacement under spinal anaesthesia. She has a history of bipolar disorder and has been on lithium for the last 2 years. Half-way through the procedure she complains of discomfort in the chest and the ECG shows irregular, broad complexes (Torsade de pointes). Her blood pressure is 100/70mmHg. Which of the following anti-arrhythmic treatment should be administered to this patient?

a. Isoprenaline infusion.
b. Intravenous lidocaine 2mg/kg.
c. Intravenous phenytoin 15mg/kg.
d. Intravenous magnesium 2g.
e. Intravenous potassium chloride.

19 A 73-year-old female was found collapsed at home. On admission to the emergency department she is confused and her core temperature is 33.2°C. Her other vital parameters are within the normal range. It is suspected that she has suffered a minor cerebrovascular event. Which of the following would be the best treatment of hypothermia in this patient?

a. Oxygen supplementation with rapid re-warming using gastric and bladder warm fluid lavage.
b. Oxygen supplementation with re-warming using warm intravenous fluid and warming blankets.
c. Intubation and ventilation and rewarming using dialysis or cardiopulmonary bypass.
d. Intubation and ventilation with rapid rewarming using gastric and bladder warm fluid lavage.
e. Intubation and ventilation with warmed intravenous fluid/warming blankets.

20 A 28-year-old female patient is scheduled for correction of kyphoscoliosis and insertion of Harrington rods. Which of the following intra-operative monitoring is most useful in detecting neurological injury during instrumentation of the spine?

a. Wake-up test.
b. Bispectral index.
c. Somatosensory evoked potentials.
d. Invasive blood pressure monitoring.
e. Peripheral nerve stimulation.

21 A 36-year-old male presents to the pain clinic with a history of pain in the left forearm associated with burning sensations, muscle spasm, swelling and discolouration. Three months before he suffered a fracture of the scaphoid bone of his left hand, which was treated surgically under general anaesthesia. The most likely diagnosis is:

a. Complex regional pain syndrome type I.
b. Post-surgical pain due to nerve damage.
c. Complex regional pain syndrome type II.
d. Peripheral vascular disease involving the upper limb.
e. Peripheral nerve injury occurring during general anaesthesia.

22 A 24-year-old man presents for extraction of two upper molar teeth under general anaesthesia. He gives a history of episodes of haemarthrosis. Blood investigations have revealed an elevated activated partial thromboplastin time (aPTT), a normal platelet count and a normal prothrombin time (PT). Which of the following haematological disorders is most likely to be present in this patient?

41

a. von Willebrand disease.
b. Haemophilia A.
c. Factor V deficiency.
d. Afibrinogenaemia.
e. Factor XIII deficiency.

23 A 50-year-old female patient presents for decompression of a thoracic epidural abscess. Her weight is 96kg and height is 158cm. She has developed increasing weakness of both lower limbs over the past 2 days. General anaesthesia is induced with propofol, atracurium and remifentanil. Soon after tracheal intubation her oxygen saturation decreases to 89%, which does not respond to increasing the inspired oxygen concentration to 100%. On auscultation bilateral equal air entry is confirmed with no added sounds. Her $EtCO_2$ decreases to 2.5kPa whilst her minute ventilation is maintained at 8L/minute. Which of these is the most likely cause of the hypoxia?

a. Pulmonary embolism.
b. Endobronchial intubation.
c. Severe bronchospasm.
d. Pulmonary oedema.
e. Air embolism.

24 A 26-year-old woman, on her first postnatal day, suffers a fit on the postnatal ward. The first step in the immediate management should be:

a. Intravenous magnesium sulphate, with a loading dose of 4g over 10 minutes.
b. Intravenous lorazepam 4mg.
c. Rapid sequence induction with thiopentone and suxamethonium.
d. Oxygen via a face mask with a reservoir bag at 15L/min.
e. Phenytoin, with a loading dose of 18mg/kg over 1 hour.

25 A 65-year-old male patient undergoing an arthroscopic procedure on the right shoulder under general anaesthesia and an interscalene block in the sitting position develops bradycardia and hypotension during the intra-operative period. The interscalene block was performed using 20ml of 1% lidocaine with epinephrine. The most appropriate treatment is:

a. Ephedrine.
b. Glycopyrrolate.
c. Atropine.
d. Metaraminol.
e. Phenylephrine.

26 A 78-year-old male presents with pain in the lower back which he has suffered for the last 2 years. The pain radiates bilaterally to the back of the thigh and groin and is increased by extension and twisting movements at the lumbar spine. The most likely cause of his pain is:

a. Discogenic lower back pain.
b. Referred pain from sacro-iliac joint arthropathy.
c. Pain due to facet joint arthropathy.
d. Pain due to spinal stenosis.
e. Pain due to muscle spasm.

27 An 84-year-old woman with rheumatoid arthritis presents for an elective cholecystectomy. At the pre-anaesthetic assessment, she describes severe neck pain with numbness and tingling in both arms. Which of the following investigations is most useful in the further management of this case?

a.   Proceed with general anaesthesia with manual in-line stabilisation.
b.   Perform lateral cervical spine X-rays.
c.   Arrange nerve conduction studies.
d.   Perform a flexion view of the cervical spine.
e.   Perform an MRI scan of the cervical spine.

28 A 35-year-old female patient with Crohn's disease presents for elective laparotomy and resection of a small bowel stricture. She has been taking 12.5mg prednisolone once a day for the last 6 months to control her disease. Which one of the following would be the most appropriate peri-operative management of her steroid treatment?

a.   Continuation only of 12.5mg prednisolone once a day.
b.   50mg intravenous hydrocortisone at induction and her usual steroid dose after surgery.
c.   Delay the surgery for 3 months.
d.   Usual steroid dose on the morning of surgery and hydrocortisone 50mg intravenously at induction, followed by 50mg three times a day by intravenous injection for 24 hours.
e.   Usual steroid dose on the morning of surgery and hydrocortisone 50mg intravenously at induction, followed by 50mg three times a day by intravenous injection for 48-72 hours.

29 A woman delivers a baby by normal vaginal delivery. A needle-through-needle combined spinal and epidural (CSE) was inserted 2 hours prior to delivery to provide labour analgesia. An initial intrathecal dose of 5µg fentanyl and 2.5mg bupivacaine was given

and nothing via the epidural component was required. Twenty-four hours after delivery, she has unilateral foot drop (no other neurology). The best course of action is:

a.   Reassurance that this is not due to the epidural.
b.   An MRI scan.
c.   A further review in 24 hours time.
d.   Immediate nerve conduction studies.
e.   A CT scan.

30 A 63-year-old male develops a brochopleural fistula following a pneumonectomy. He is ventilated on the ICU, but achieving adequate tidal volume is proving to be difficult due to an air leak of 2.5L/min through the fistula. Which one of the following would be most effective in achieving adequate ventilation in this patient?

a.   Adding PEEP of 7.5cm of H_2O.
b.   Decreasing the inflation pressure.
c.   Increasing the flow rate by 2.5L/min.
d.   High frequency jet ventilation.
e.   Decreasing the respiratory rate.

Set 2 answers

1   Answer: B. Intravenous DDAVP.

Diabetes insipidus is the common endocrine dysfunction following trans-sphenoidal hypophysectomy. The diagnosis of diabetes insipidus is supported by a high urine output, low serum osmolarity and low specific gravity of the urine. Other causes of high urine output include diuresis secondary to hyperglycaemia, mannitol or crystalloid administration. Neurogenic diabetes insipidus should be treated with 5 units of aqueous vasopressin subcutaneously or 2-4mg of DDAVP (1-desamino 8-D arginine vasopressin) I.V. or S.C. In neurogenic diabetes insipidus, urine osmolarity increases following administration of vasopressin or DDAVP.

Further reading
1. Cronin AJ. Acute postcraniotomy agitation. In: *Near misses in neuroanaesthesia*. Russell GB, Cronin AJ, Longo S, Blackburn TW, Eds. Butterworth Heinemann, 2002; Case 43: 155-7.
2. Osborn IP. Trans-sphenoidal hypophysectomy. In: *Clinical cases in anaesthesia*, 3rd ed. Reed AP, Yudkowitz FS, Eds. Philadelphia, USA: Elsevier Churchill Livingstone, 2005; Case 22: 113-6.

2   Answer: D. Helical CT with sagittal reformat.

Although lateral and anteroposterior cervical spine X-rays with an open mouth view have been considered 'gold standards' for the exclusion of c-spine injury, they can miss a substantial amount of bony and soft tissue injury. An MRI scan can detect soft tissue injury but may miss bony lesions on the posterior wall of the cervical spine. Helical CT with sagittal reconstruction is the best way to exclude cervical spine injury. Dynamic fluoroscopy involves passive manipulation of the cervical spine under real-time fluoroscopic imaging. It has a low sensitivity and a false negative rate of 0.33%. There is no conclusive evidence for the use of dynamic fluoroscopy as a screening test for cervical spine injury.

Further reading
1. Bonhomme V, Hans P. Management of the unstable cervical spine: elective versus emergency cases. *Current Opinions in Anesthesiology* 2009; 22: 579-85.
2. Richards PJ. Cervical spine clearance: a review. *Injury* 2005; 36: 248-69.

46

3 Answer: E. Tension pneumothorax.

Pneumothorax is one of the complications which can follow central venous cannulation. Severe bronchospasm is an alternative diagnosis. The clinical history, however, with a difficult central line insertion, is suggestive of a tension pneumothorax. Anaphylaxis may present with similar clinical features of tachycardia, hypotension and increased airway pressure, but is most likely to occur at induction or following a particular drug administration.

Further reading
1. Giacomini M, Iapichino M, Armani S, *et al.* How to avoid and manage pneumothorax. *Vascular Access* 2006; 7: 7-14.

4 Answer: A. Intrinsic renal failure.

The history and blood/urine results indicate that this patient is in renal failure. In intrinsic renal failure, the tubules are dysfunctional and therefore electrolytes and water are not absorbed efficiently. This leads to dilute urine with an osmolarity of less than 300mosmol/L and urine Na⁺ loss of more than 20mmol/L.

In pre-renal failure, renal tubules still work efficiently and therefore all the unwanted elements are excreted in the minimum possible volume in order to conserve water. This leads to very concentrated urine (high specific gravity >1.020, urine osmolarity >500). The tubules also absorb most of the filtered Na^+ and urine Na^+ is <20mmol/L. Both urea and creatinine are excreted in a small volume of urine and therefore the urine: plasma creatinine ratio is >40 and for urea >20.

Further reading

1. *Anaesthesia and intensive care A-Z. An encyclopaedia of principles and practice*, 4th ed. Yentis SM, Hirsch NP, Smith GB. Oxford, UK: Butterworth-Heinemann, 2009: 473-4.

5   Answer: C. Nephrogenic diabetes insipidus.

47

Diabetes insipidus (DI) can be classified as central or nephrogenic. Central DI is caused by reduced or absent synthesis or release of antidiuretic hormone (ADH, vasopressin), whereas nephrogenic DI is caused by the reduced responsiveness of distal tubules and collecting ducts to ADH.

A common side effect of lithium is nephrogenic DI; about one third of patients on long-term lithium develop diabetes insipidus. Lithium may reduce the number of ADH-regulated water channels (aquaporin-2) in the collecting ducts, thereby reducing water absorption in the distal tubules with resulting polyuria and polydypsia.

Rhabdomyolysis due to associated crush injury may result in acute renal failure and low urine output. Urine testing is positive for blood and myoglobin. Bendrofluazide can cause a diuresis but is unlikely to cause such a marked polyuria as this. Gentamicin, an aminoglycoside antibiotic, can cause impaired renal function.

Further reading

1. Paw H, Slingo ME, Tinker M. Late onset of nephrogenic diabetes inspidus following cessation of lithium therapy. *Anesthesia Intensive Care* 2007; 35: 278-80.

6   Answer: C. Arrange for an MRI scan of the spine.

The clinical triad of fever, back pain, and neurologic deficit is suggestive of an epidural abscess. A sequential evolution of symptoms and signs has been described, with localised spinal pain, radicular pain and paresthesiae, muscular weakness, sensory loss, sphincter dysfunction, and, finally, paralysis. The incidence is extremely rare but is partly affected by the time the epidural catheter has been *in situ*, and the general health of the patient. In order to prevent permanent neurological sequelae, an early definitive diagnosis by MRI scan and surgical decompression of the spinal cord and drainage of the abscess is essential. Consultation with a neurosurgeon or spinal surgeon should be requested when a spinal epidural abscess is detected or strongly suspected. Increasing neurological deficit, persistent severe pain, or persistent fever and leukocytosis are all indications for surgery.

Further reading
1. Grewal S, Hocking G, Wildsmith JA. Epidural abscesses. *British Journal of Anaesthesia* 2006; 96: 292-302.

7   Answer: E. Electromyography.

Nerve conduction studies include tests for both sensory and motor components. The likely cause for weakness of the foot in this patient is compression of the common peroneal nerve by the lithotomy leg holder. A detailed history and complete neurological examination is essential prior to any investigations.

Injury to the common peroneal nerve causes foot drop and loss of sensation over the dorsum of the foot. Electromyography involves recording the electrical activity in the muscle. It is useful in distinguishing peripheral neuropathy from nerve root compression from a more central cause and establishing the site of the lesion. The other differential diagnosis includes a lumbar disc prolapse causing nerve root compression for which CT and MRI scans are useful investigations. Spontaneous foot drop in a previously healthy patient may be due to a metabolic cause such as diabetes mellitus.

Further reading

1. Yigit NA, Bagbanc B, Celebi H. Drop foot after pediatric urological surgery under general and epidural anesthesia. *Anesth Analg* 2006; 103: 1616.
2. Horlocker TT, Cabanela ME, Wedel DJ. Does postoperative epidural analgesia increase the risk of peroneal nerve palsy after total knee arthroplasty? *Anesth Analg* 1994; 79: 495-500.
3. Hubbert CH. Peroneal palsy after epidural analgesia. *Anesth Analg* 1993; 77: 405-6.
4. Hogan QH. Pathophysiology of peripheral nerve injury during regional anesthesia. *Reg Anesth Pain Med* 2008; 33: 435-41.

8   Answer: B. ST-T wave abnormalities.

In about 50% of patients with ischaemic heart disease, the ECG may be normal. ST-T wave abnormalities are the most commonly observed ECG findings (65-90%). Tall R waves in V5 and V6, and deep S waves in lead V1 indicate left ventricular hypertrophy which may be seen in 10-20% of abnormal ECGs. Pathological Q waves account for 0.5 to 8% of ECG abnormalities.

Further reading

1. Mittnacht A, Reich DL. Recent myocardial infarction. In: *Clinical cases in anaesthesia*, 3rd ed. Reed AP, Yudkowitz FS, Eds. Philadelphia, USA: Elsevier Churchill Livingstone, 2005; Case 3: 15-20.

9   Answer: A. Biliary tract ultrasound.

This patient is displaying the signs and symptoms of acute pancreatitis, supported by the blood results. Biliary tract ultrasound is recommended in the initial assessment of all cases of acute pancreatitis. It is non-invasive, relatively inexpensive and may be performed at the bedside. The sensitivity of this study in detecting pancreatitis is 62 to 95%. A CT scan is indicated if the diagnosis is equivocal, to rule out alternative intra-abdominal catastrophes, and to detect and stage regional complications such as pancreatic necrosis. If the diagnosis is clear, it may be appropriate to delay CT imaging for at least 48-72 hours after the onset of symptoms because the full extent of pancreatic necrosis cannot be determined until this time. A contrast-enhanced CT scan is useful to assess the severity by detecting pancreatic necrosis and the degree of peri-pancreatic collection. A plain X-ray of the abdomen may show a gas-filled duodenum secondary to obstruction, but this is not a specific diagnostic test.

Further reading

1. Young SP, Thompson JP. Severe acute pancreatitis. *British Journal of Anaesthesia CEACCP* 2008; 8: 125-8.

10 Answer: B. D-Dimer.

Fibrinolysis is an important component of disseminated intravascular coagulation (DIC). Breakdown products of fibrin, fibrin degradation products (FDPs) and D-Dimers are therefore elevated. The specificity of these tests is, however, limited because other conditions such as venous thrombo-embolism, trauma and recent surgery can lead to elevated FDPs and D-Dimers. The ongoing consumption of coagulation factors leads to elevated global clotting times (aPTT and PT). The diagnosis of DIC should be based on both clinical history and laboratory tests. The laboratory tests include FDPs, D-Dimers, fibrinogen level, PT and aPTT. D-Dimers would not be elevated in dilutional coagulopathy.

Further reading

1. Becker JU, Wira CR. Disseminated intravascular coagulation: differential diagnosis and workup. (http://emedicine.medscape.com/article/779097-diagnosis).

11 Answer: C. Epidural steroid injection.

Sciatica is defined as the pain caused by compression or irritation of the sciatic nerve or one of the five nerve roots from which it originates. The pain is felt in the lower back, buttock, posterior aspect of the thigh, or posterolaterally in the leg and foot. The patient may experience numbness, muscular weakness, pins and needles or tingling. Sciatica can be caused by various factors. If caused by lumbar disc prolapse or herniation, it will resolve in about 90% of patients over a few weeks with no specific intervention. Persistent sciatica pain can be treated with different modalities. These include simple analgesics such as paracetamol and NSAIDs, sodium and calcium channel blockers, tricyclic antidepressants, opioids, physiotherapy, epidural steroids, and surgical intervention. Evidence of effectiveness for these measures is, however, limited. Surgery speeds up the resolution of pain; however, 2 years post-surgery, outcomes are equivalent, so patient preference is an important factor when deciding treatment. Long-term bed rest as a treatment in sciatica is rarely practised conservative treatment nowadays and, commonly, patients are advised bed rest for a few days only. In this patient, as he is a lorry driver, it would be wise to avoid strong opioids if possible as these could affect his driving. Epidural steroids are used in the treatment of sciatica with limited effectiveness.

Further reading
1. Gregory DS, Seto CK, Wortley GC, Shugart CM. Acute lumbar disk pain: navigating evaluation and treatment choices. *Am Fam Physician* 2008; 78: 835-42.

12   Answer: B. MRI scan of the cervical spine.

This patient has had a parathyroidectomy. During surgical positioning, the neck is usually hyper-extended to improve surgical access. In a patient with pre-existing cervical spine disease, such as disc prolapse and spinal canal stenosis, extension manoeuvres during laryngoscopy and positioning may damage the spinal cord leading to tetraparesis. Patients with chronic renal failure are prone to degenerative disease of the spinal cord. In addition, extradural deposition of amyloid is seen in patients on long-term dialysis which can result in spinal canal stenosis.

The neurological symptoms of hypocalcaemia include numbness, a tingling sensation in the peri-oral area and fingers and toes, muscle cramps and carpopedal spasm (tetany). Hypocalcaemia following parathyroidectomy usually occurs 12-24 hours after surgery. A CT scan of the head would be useful in assessing intracranial lesions, but would not identify lesions of the cervical spine, which would be best identified with an MRI of the spine itself.

Further reading
1. Mercieri M, Paolini S, *et al.* Tetraplegia following parathyroidectomy in two long-term haemodialysis patients. *Anaesthesia* 2009; 64: 1010-3.
2. Whiteson JH, Panaro N, *et al.* Tetraparesis following dental extraction: case report and discussion of preventive measures for cervical spinal hyperextension injury. *The Journal of Spinal Cord Medicine* 1997; 20: 422-5.
3. Mihai R, Farndon JR. Parathyroid disease and calcium metabolism. *British Journal of Anaesthesia* 2000; 85: 29-43.

13   Answer: D. Metabolic alkalosis with acidic urine.

Infantile pyloric stenosis is a medical emergency requiring surgical intervention for definitive treatment. It usually presents between the 3rd and 5th week of life and is more common in males (M:F 4:1). Projectile vomiting causes loss of K^+, H^+, Cl^-, Na^+ and water, leading to metabolic alkalosis. Initially, alkaline urine is produced as excess plasma bicarbonate is excreted. If severe volume depletion occurs with continuing vomiting, the kidney conserves Na^+ (and water) in exchange for H^+ and K^+ ions. This causes 'paradoxical' acid urine in the presence of metabolic alkalosis.

Further reading
1. Fell D, Chelliah S. Infantile pyloric stenosis. *British Journal of Anaesthesia CEPD review* 2001; 1: 85-8.

14   Answer: C. Transcranial Doppler.

Stroke is the most common major complication of carotid endarterectomy (CEA). Embolisation of thrombus or air during manipulation is the most likely cause of cerebral ischaemia. Transcranial Doppler measures the blood flow velocity in the middle cerebral artery on the operative side. It is an extremely sensitive detector of cerebral embolisation.

Electro-encephalography (EEG) is the most sensitive method for the detection of cerebral ischaemia in the unconscious patient, demonstrated by changes such as reduced amplitude, decreased frequency and burst suppression. Intra-operative EEG monitoring is, however, too complex to use in a theatre environment and requires specialist experience to interpret the findings. A unilateral decrease in amplitude and an increase in latency of somatosensory evoked potentials (SSEP) indicate ischaemia, but SSEP are less sensitive than EEG for detecting ischaemia.

Further reading

1. Schwartz AE. Carotid endarterectomy. In: *Clinical cases in anaesthesia*, 3rd ed. Reed AP, Yudkowitz FS, Eds. Philadelphia, USA: Elsevier Churchill Livingstone, 2005; Case 19: 101-3.
2. Babikian VL, Cantelmo NL. Cerebrovascular monitoring during carotid endarterectomy. *Stroke* 2000; 31: 1799-1801.

15 Answer: D. Pulmonary function tests to estimate postoperative FEV1.

A joint initiative by the British Thoracic Society and the Society of Cardiothoracic Surgeons of Great Britain and Ireland (SCTS) has produced detailed recommendations for the selection and management of patients with potentially operable lung cancer. According to these, the pulmonary function of the patient undergoing pneumonectomy should be assessed as follows:

♦ No further respiratory function tests are required in patients undergoing pneumonectomy if the post-bronchodilator FEV1 is >2.0L, provided that there is no evidence of interstitial lung disease or unexpected disability due to shortness of breath.
♦ All patients with a post-bronchodilator FEV1 <2.0L should have:
  • full pulmonary function tests including estimation of the transfer factor for carbon monoxide (TLCO);
  • measurement of oxygen saturation on air at rest;
  • a quantitative isotope perfusion scan.
♦ Estimated postoperative FEV1 >40% of predicted and estimated postoperative TLCO >40% of predicted and oxygen saturation (SaO_2) >90% on air indicates average risk.
♦ Estimated postoperative FEV1 <40% of predicted and estimated postoperative TLCO <40% of predicted indicates high risk.

Further reading

1. https://www.brit-thoracic.org.uk/Portals/0/Clinical%20Information/Lung%20Cancer/Guidelines/lungcancersurgery.pdf.

16 Answer: D. Morphine 100µg/kg as an intravenous bolus.

This child needs treatment of his pain as soon as possible. A morphine bolus is the most appropriate as the onset time of pain relief will be shorter than most of the other mentioned options. Intramuscular codeine is painful and its slower onset may make it inadequate. Performing an axillary plexus block in a distressed child is not an ideal option; it has a delayed onset and potential for failure. Although entonox has a rapid onset of action it may be difficult to administer and only lasts for a short time. It may also cause dizziness, nausea and vomiting. Pain after open reduction of a fracture in children can usually be adequately managed by regular paracetamol and ibuprofen with PRN Oramorph. A morphine infusion is rarely needed and would require a bolus prior to its administration.

Further reading
1. Webber SJ, Barker I. Paediatric anaesthetic pharmacology. *British Journal of Anaesthesia CEPD review* 2003; 3: 50-3.

17 Answer: B. Intravenous saline and furosemide.

Hypercalcaemia most commonly occurs due to either malignancy or primary hyperparathyroidism. The normal range of serum calcium levels is 2.1 to 2.5mmol/L. Approximately 40% of calcium is bound to albumin, 50% is ionised and is in the physiologically active form, and the remaining 10% forms complexes with anions. Plasma calcium is regulated by parathyroid hormone (PTH), vitamin D and calcitonin. Calcium enters the body through the small intestine and is eventually excreted via the kidney. Bone can act as a storage depot. This entire system is controlled through a feedback loop; individual hormones respond as needed to increase or decrease the serum calcium concentration.

The initial step in the treatment of hypercalcaemia is hydration with saline; this helps to decrease the calcium level by dilution. The expansion of extracellular volume also increases renal calcium clearance. Loop diuretics may be used in conjunction with intravenous hydration to increase calcium excretion. This may also prevent volume overload during the therapy. The rate of fluid therapy depends on the degree of hypercalcaemia, severity of dehydration, and the ability of the patient to tolerate rehydration. Haemodialysis may be necessary to correct hypercalcaemia in patients with renal failure.

Intravenous bisphosphates and calcitonin should be considered for the management of symptomatic hypercalcaemia. Corticosteroids tend to be more effective in patients with hypercalcaemia due to myeloma, sarcoidosis and vitamin D excess.

Further reading
1. Ariyan CE, Sosa JA. Assessment and management of patients with abnormal calcium. *Crit Care Med* 2004; 32: S146-54.
2. Mihai R, Farndon JR. Parathyroid disease and calcium metabolism. *British Journal of Anaesthesia* 2000; 85: 29-43.

18 Answer: D. Intravenous magnesium 2g.

Torsade de pointes is a type of ventricular tachycardia in which the morphology of the QRS complexes varies from beat to beat. The ventricular rate can vary between 150 to 250 beats per minute. The definition also requires that the QT interval be increased markedly (usually to 600msec or greater). The underlying basis for rhythm disturbance is a delay in phase III of the action potential.

Prolongation of the QT interval may be congenital (e.g. Romano Ward syndrome). The acquired conditions that predispose to Torsade de pointes are hypokalaemia, hypomagnesaemia, cirrhosis and hypothyroidism. Some drugs can prolong the QT interval; these include phenothiazines, tricyclic antidepressants, lithium carbonate, cisapride, highly active antiretrovirals, some fluoroquinolones, and any other drugs using the CYP3A metabolic pathway. Risk factors for this condition are female gender, history of syncope, congenital deafness and a family history of sudden death.

Magnesium is the treatment of choice for Torsade de pointes and is effective even in a patient with a normal magnesium level. Other therapies include overdrive pacing and isoprenaline infusion. A patient with unstable blood pressure should be treated with electrical cardioversion or defibrillation. Anecdotal evidence exists for successful conversion with phenytoin and lidocaine.

Further reading

1. Roden DM. A practical approach to Torsade de pointes. *Clin Cardiol* 1997; 20: 285-90.
2. Schenck JB, Rizvi AA, Lin T. Severe primary hypothyroidism manifesting with Torsades de pointes. *Am J Med Sci* 2006; 331: 154-6.

19 Answer: B. Oxygen supplementation with rewarming using warm intravenous fluid and warming blankets.

The body's core temperature is closely regulated between 37.2°C +/- 0.4°C. The body maintains a stable core temperature by balancing heat production and heat loss. The hypothalamus controls thermoregulation via increased heat conservation (peripheral vasoconstriction, and behavioural responses) and heat production (shivering, and increasing levels of thyroxine and epinephrine). Depending on body temperature, hypothermia can be graded as mild hypothermia (32-35°C), moderate hypothermia (28-32°C), and severe hypothermia (<28°C).

Treatment depends on the degree of hypothermia. Patients with mild hypothermia may be rewarmed using commonly available measures (warm I.V. fluids, warm blankets, removal of cold, wet clothing). Since the risk of cardiac dysrhythmia is low, surface rewarming is adequate. In severe hypothermia, the risk of cardiac arrhythmias is high and the treatment is aimed at maintaining or restoring cardiac perfusion and maximising oxygenation until the core temperature is at least 30°C.

Further reading

1. Polderman KH. Mechanisms of action, physiological effects, and complications of hypothermia. *Crit Care Med* 2009; 37: S186-202.
2. Management of inadvertent hypothermia, NICE clinical guideline. (http://www.nice.org.uk/CG65).
3. Kirkbride DA, Buggy DJ. Thermoregulation and mild peri-operative hypothermia. *British Journal of Anaesthesia CEPD review* 2003; 3: 24-8.
4. Kirkpatrick AW, Chun R, Brown R, *et al.* Hypothermia and the trauma patient. *Canadian Journal of Surgery* 1999; 42: 333-43.

20 Answer: C. Somatosensory evoked potentials.

The 'wake-up' test involves reducing the depth of anaesthesia to a plane where the patient can respond to simple commands in order to assess motor function. The anaesthetic is then deepened to allow completion of the surgical procedure. Disadvantages include coughing, bucking and the risk of accidental extubation during this wake-up period.

The bispectral index monitors the depth of anaesthesia. It is not specific to this surgical procedure but is useful in situations where awareness is a significant risk. Invasive blood pressure monitoring and peripheral nerve stimulation are the essential components of monitoring during the above procedure but are not specific to the detection of nerve injury.

Continuous intra-operative neurophysiological monitoring includes somatosensory evoked potentials (SSEP) and motor evoked potentials (MEP). SSEP involves stimulating peripheral nerves and detecting the response with epidural or scalp electrodes. Decreased amplitude and increased latency indicate nerve injury. SSEPs are useful to avoid spinal cord damage during insertion of Harrington rods, a specific complication related to this operation. MEP involves using a transcranial impulse to stimulate the motor cortex; the resulting signal is detected as compound muscle action potentials. MEPs are more challenging to apply and often require the use of TIVA with minimal or no muscle relaxants. Inhalational and intravenous anaesthetic agents can cause a significant decrease in the amplitude or latency of MEPs. A combination of an opioid, such as a remifentanil infusion, and a low dose of propofol is a particularly successful technique during the monitoring of MEPs.

Further reading
1. Osborn IP, Spine surgery. In: *Clinical cases in anaesthesia*, 3rd ed. Reed AP, Yudkowitz FS, Eds. Philadelphia, USA: Elsevier Churchill Livingstone, 2005; Case 21: 109-22.
2. Entwistle MA, Patel D. Scoliosis surgery in children. *British Journal of Anaesthesia CEACCP* 2006; 6: 13-6.

21   Answer: A. Complex regional pain syndrome type I.

Complex regional pain syndrome (CRPS) type I consists of continuous pain in the extremity following trauma, including fractures. The pain does not, however, correspond to a particular dermatome. The pain is increased with movement and patients often complain of cool, clammy skin which later becomes pale, cold, stiff and atrophied. Many patients with CRPS will exhibit some type of movement disorder ranging from reduced strength to tremor, myoclonus and dystonia.

CRPS II consists of pain and the symptoms described above in the distribution of a partially damaged peripheral nerve. The clinical features and management of CRPS I and CRPS II are similar. The only difference between the two types is the presence of a definable nerve injury in CRPS II.

The International Association for the Study of Pain (IASP) lists the following diagnostic criteria for complex regional pain syndrome I (CRPS I):

- The presence of an initiating noxious event or a cause of immobilization.
- Continuing pain, allodynia (perception of pain from a non-painful stimulus), or hyperalgesia disproportionate to the initiating event.
- Evidence of changes in skin blood flow, or abnormal sudomotor activity in the area of pain.
- The diagnosis is excluded by the existence of any condition that would otherwise account for the degree of pain and dysfunction.

Further reading
1. Wilson JG, Serpell MG. Complex regional pain syndrome. *British Journal of Anaesthesia CEACCP* 2007; 7: 51-4.

22   Answer: B. Haemophilia A.

Haemophilia A is the most common hereditary coagulation disorder. It is due to deficiency of Factor VIII and primarily affects males. Haemophilia A may present with haemarthrosis, bruising occurring easily, and potentially fatal haemorrhage following trauma and surgery. PT and platelet counts are normal but the aPTT is prolonged. Patients with severe haemophilia have Factor VIII levels less than 1% of normal.

von Willebrand's disease occurs due to the deficiency of von Willebrand Factor, which is necessary for the adherence of platelets to the exposed endothelium. The bleeding time is prolonged but the platelet count is normal. The clinical presentation includes bruising readily and bleeding from the mucosal surfaces (epistaxis).

In Factor V deficiency, PT, PTT and bleeding times are all prolonged. The bleeding is most often from the mucosal membranes.

Afibrinogenaemia is due to congenital absence of fibrinogen. Coagulation tests such as bleeding time, PT, PTT and thrombin time are usually prolonged.

Further reading
1. Coagulopathies. In: *Anesthesia and co-existing disease*, 4th ed. Stoelting RK, Dierdorf SF. Philadelphia, USA: Churchill Livingstone, 2002; 489-504.

23 Answer: A. Pulmonary embolism.

This patient is obese and suffers with immobility due to paraparesis; both are risk factors for pulmonary embolism. The causes of desaturation should be systematically considered starting from the anaesthetic machine all the way to the lungs. Once the oxygen delivery, integrity of the breathing system and airway patency are confirmed, any cause arising in the cardiorespiratory system, such as bronchospasm, pneumothorax, and endobronchial intubation should be diagnosed and corrected. In this scenario desaturation is associated with a low $EtCO_2$. Other causes of low $EtCO_2$, such as breathing system disconnection, a leak in the gas sampling line and hyperventilation, should be ruled out.

Clinical examination has ruled out the two common causes, bronchospasm and endobronchial intubation, and also confirmed the correct placement of the endotracheal tube. The most likely cause is ventilation and perfusion mismatch, which would be a pulmonary embolism.

Further reading

1. Riedel M. Diagnosing pulmonary embolism. *Postgraduate Medical Journal* 2004; 80: 309-19.
2. van Beek EJR, Elliot CA, Kiely DG. Diagnosis and initial treatment of patients with suspected pulmonary thromboembolism. *British Journal of Anaesthesia CEACCP* 2009; 9(4): 119-24.

24 Answer: D. Oxygen via a face mask with a reservoir bag at 15L/min.

Although magnesium sulphate is the treatment of choice for eclampsia, it is most important to administer oxygen immediately before implementing other therapy. Do not leave the woman alone but call for help, including a senior obstetrician. Ensure that it is safe to approach the woman and aim to prevent maternal injury during the convulsion. Place the woman in the left lateral position and administer oxygen. Assess the airway and breathing and check the pulse and blood pressure. Benzodiazepines and phenytoin should no longer be used as first-line drugs. A loading dose of 4g of magnesium should be administered by an infusion pump over 5-10 minutes, followed by a further infusion of 1g/hour, maintained for 24 hours following the most recent seizure. Recurrent seizures should be treated with a further bolus of 2g of magnesium sulphate.

Further reading

1. RCOG Green-Top 10A guideline: The management of severe pre-eclampsia/eclampsia (www.rcog.org.uk).
2. The Eclampsia Trial Collaborative Group: Which anticonvulsant for women with eclampsia? Evidence from the Collaborative Eclampsia Trial. *Lancet* 1995; 345: 1455-63.

25 Answer: A. Ephedrine.

This is likely to be the Bezold-Jarisch reflex (BJR), a paradoxical activation of the left ventricular mechanoreceptors caused by reduced venous return, due to pooling of blood in the lower extremities in the sitting position. Ephedrine is the drug of choice. It is a sympathomimetic amine with both α and β effects. Via its β1 effects it causes positive chronotropy and inotropy which increases cardiac output, and through its α1 effects it causes peripheral vasoconstriction. Phenylephrine has predominantly α1 effects causing peripheral vasoconstriction. Metaraminol is also a potent vasoconstrictor. Both phenylephrine and metaraminol will increase blood pressure and can cause reflex bradycardia. Atropine alone is not effective in treating this condition.

BJR, with bradycardia and hypotension, may progress to cardiovascular collapse, and is most commonly seen during surgery on the shoulder performed under an interscalene block in the sitting position. Peripheral vasodilatation, increased contractility from absorbed epinephrine and vigorous contractions of a relatively empty ventricle are three components that may contribute to BJR.

Further reading

1. Campagna JA, Carter C. Clinical relevance of the Bezold-Jarisch reflex. *Anesthesiology* 2003; 98: 1250-60.
2. Reiss LWJ. Brachial plexus anesthesia. In: *Clinical cases in anaesthesia*, 3rd ed. Reed AP, Yudkowitz FS, Eds. Philadelphia, USA: Elsevier Churchill Livingstone, 2005; Case 57: 337.

26 Answer: C. Pain due to facet joint arthropathy.

Low back pain (LBP) is a common musculoskeletal complaint, with a reported lifetime incidence of 60-90%. Various structures have been suggested as possible sources of chronic LBP and these include the posterior longitudinal ligament, dorsal root ganglia, dura, annular fibres, muscles of the lumbar spine, and the facet joints. Two medial branches of the dorsal rami innervate the facet joints. The presence of nociceptive nerve fibres in the various tissue structures of facet joints suggests that these structures may cause pain when placed under increased or abnormal loads. Biomechanically, facet joints assume a prominent role in resisting stress. During the rotation of the spine, the facet capsular ligaments protect the intervertebral discs by preventing excessive movement. There are no unique signs or symptoms identified which can help in diagnosing the pain originating from the facet joint. However, biomechanical studies of the facet joint during extension and rotation support the belief that facet joint pain is worse with extension and rotation. Lumbar facet joint pain is lateralised and can radiate to the groin and thigh.

Further reading

1. Manchikanti L, Boswell MV, Singh V, et al. Prevalence of facet joint pain in chronic spinal pain of cervical, thoracic, and lumbar regions. BMC Musculoskelet Disord 2004; 5: 15.

27 Answer: E. Perform an MRI scan of the cervical spine.

These symptoms in a chronic rheumatoid patient with possible erosive disease are suggestive of atlanto-axial subluxation with spinal cord compromise. Associated symptoms include occipital headaches and motor weakness. Direct laryngoscopy and tracheal intubation may cause irreversible spinal cord damage if there is ligamentous instability. Elective surgery should be delayed and further investigations organised to confirm the diagnosis. Flexion and extension cervical spine X-rays demonstrate the subluxation and are the most appropriate initial investigation. However, in a patient with significant symptoms, an MRI scan provides more details, such as nerve root compression, spinal cord compression and spinal canal involvement. It may be necessary to arrange spinal stabilisation surgery prior to any other elective surgery. If the patient presents for emergency surgery, these investigations may not be possible, and the cervical spine should be treated as unstable.

Further reading

1. Fombon F, Thompson J. Anaesthesia for the adult patient with rheumatoid arthritis. British Journal of Anaesthesia CEACCP 2006; 6: 235-39.

28 Answer: E. Usual steroid dose on the morning of surgery and hydrocortisone 50mg intravenously at induction, followed by 50mg three times a day by intravenous injection for 48-72 hours.

This patient is scheduled to have major elective surgery. During prolonged therapy with corticosteroids, adrenal atrophy develops. Abrupt withdrawal can lead to acute adrenal insufficiency. To compensate for diminished adrenocortical response caused by prolonged corticosteroid treatment, any significant intercurrent illness, trauma or surgical procedures, there should be a temporary increase in the dose. The *British National Formulary* recommends the following regimen for corticosteroid replacement in patients who have taken more than 10mg prednisolone daily (or equivalent) within 3 months of surgery:

♦ Minor surgery: usual oral corticosteroid dose on the morning of surgery or hydrocortisone 25-50mg intravenously at induction; the usual oral corticosteroid dose is recommenced after surgery.
♦ Moderate or major surgery: usual oral corticosteroid dose on the morning of surgery and hydrocortisone 25-50mg intravenously at induction, followed by hydrocortisone 25-50mg three times a day by intravenous injection for 24 hours after moderate surgery or for 48-72 hours after major surgery; the usual pre-operative oral corticosteroid dose is recommenced on stopping hydrocortisone injections.

Further reading

1. Joint Formulary Committee. *British National Formulary*, 58th ed. London: British Medical Association and Royal Pharmaceutical Society of Great Britain; 2009.
2. Davies M, Hardman J. Anaesthesia and adrenocortical disease. *British Journal of Anaesthesia CEACCP* 2005; 5: 122-6.
3. Nicholson G, Burrin JM, Hall GM. Peri-operative steroid supplementation. *Anaesthesia* 1998; 53: 1091-104.

29 Answer: B. An MRI scan.

Unilateral foot drop may be the only presenting symptom of conus injury and a needle-through-needle technique for CSE technique carries a risk of this problem occurring. A CT scan is not the best imaging technique to look for this problem, so an MRI scan is indicated. Other pathologies which can cause foot drop in this situation include disc prolapse and space-occupying lesions (though other neurological signs and symptoms are more likely to be present with the latter). If the MRI scan is normal further management should include referral to a neurologist and possible nerve conduction studies.

Further reading
1. Reynolds F. Damage to the conus medullaris following spinal anaesthesia. *Anaesthesia* 2001; 56: 235-47.
2. Complications of obstetric regional anaesthesia. In: *Complications of regional anaesthesia*, 2nd ed. Finucane BT, Ed. Springer, 2007: Chapter 14.

30 Answer: D. High frequency jet ventilation.

Bronchopleural fistula can occur after a pneumonectomy due to the failure of the bronchial stump to heal. As the bronchus is in direct connection with the pleural cavity, some of the tidal volume is lost into the pleural cavity affecting achievable lung ventilation. Management of a ventilated patient with a bronchopleural fistula is particularly challenging and it is often difficult to wean a patient from the ventilator. High frequency ventilation with small tidal volumes, low airway pressure and a high respiratory rate provides the best chance of ventilating the lungs in these patients if conventional ventilation fails.

Further reading
1. Lois N, Noppen M. Bronchopleural fistulas: an overview of the problem with special focus on endoscopic management. *Chest* 2005; 128: 3955-65.

Set 3 questions

1   A 50-year-old man with Parkinson's disease is suffering from severe
    postoperative nausea and vomiting following an inguinal hernia
    repair under general anaesthesia. The most suitable choice of anti-
    emetic from this list for this patient would be:

a.   Intravenous metoclopramide 10mg.
b.   Intravenous dexamethasone 8mg.
c.   Intramuscular prochlorperazine 12.5mg.
d.   Intravenous droperidol 12.5mg.
e.   Intravenous ondansetron 4mg.

2   A 64-year-old female is brought to the emergency department after
    being stabbed in the groin. She is comatose, her BP is 68/34, pulse
    120 bpm and she is very pale. Her haemoglobin is 4.5g/dL. There
    is ST depression on a 12-lead ECG. She is wearing a bracelet
    which states 'Jehovah's Witness'. There is no other information
    available. The most appropriate management to treat her
    hypovolaemia would be:

a.   Start immediate cell salvage via a 'closed circuit'.
b.   Administer intravenous iron.
c.   Transfuse 4 units of O-negative allogenic blood.
d.   Try to contact the next-of-kin.
e.   Give 500ml of Gelofusin.

3

An anaesthetist administers 10ml of 0.5% bupivacaine as part of an epidural top-up for a Caesarean section. One minute after completing the injection, the patient complains of dizziness, difficulty in breathing and then starts to convulse. She then suffers a VF cardiac arrest. The most appropriate management in the first 4 minutes would be:

a. Defibrillation, CPR, adrenaline, amiodarone.
b. Defibrillation, CPR, adrenaline, Caesarean section.
c. CPR, adrenaline, 20% Intralipid, Caesarean section.
d. CPR, defibrillation, 20% Intralipid, Caesarean section.
e. CPR, defibrillation, adrenaline, 20% Intralipid.

4

A 54-year-old man has suffered a flu-like illness which has lasted 3 days. Ten days later he presented with worsening bilateral leg weakness which progressed over the next few days to involve his upper limbs. He was admitted to the intensive care unit with a diagnosis of Guillain-Barré syndrome. Which of the following interventions is likely to have the best disease-modifying effect in his case?

a. Non-invasive ventilation.
b. Corticosteroid therapy.
c. Intravenous immunoglobulin given over 5 days.
d. CSF filtration.
e. Physiotherapy.

5

A woman with HELLP syndrome requires a Caesarean section urgently. Her platelet count 12 hours ago was 96 x 10^9/L and has now dropped to 65 x 10^9/L. The other blood investigation results are Hb 8.2g/dL, WBC 15 x 10^9/L, bilirubin 45µmol/L, ALT 150IU/L, INR 1.7, and APTT 1.9. Her BP is 140/100mmHg following treatment with labetalol and magnesium sulphate. Which one of the following is the best anaesthetic option?

a. Single-shot spinal anaesthesia.
b. Platelet transfusion, followed by single-shot spinal anaesthesia.
c. Epidural anaesthesia.
d. Combined spinal-epidural anaesthesia.
e. General anaesthesia with attenuation of the response to laryngoscopy and intubation.

6 A 62-year-old female with widespread metastatic carcinoma of the rectum is on morphine sulphate (MST) 200mg b.d., gabapentin 600mg t.d.s., paracetamol 1g q.d.s. and Oramorph 40mg 4-hourly. More recently her pain control has been poor, needing an increase in the dose of MST. Although this has relieved her pain it has caused unacceptable side effects. Her life expectancy is about 2 years. Which of the following would be most likely to improve her pain control with minimal risk of side effects?

a. Epidural infusion of opioids via a tunnelled catheter.
b. Intrathecal opioid delivery via an implanted pump.
c. Transdermal fentanyl patches.
d. Sublingual buprenorphine 0.4mg added to the existing analgesia.
e. Increasing the frequency of administration of MST.

7 A 35-year-old female underwent bilateral endoscopic thoracic sympathectomy for palmar hyperhydrosis. Which of the following complications is most likely to occur in the postoperative period?

a. Compensatory sweating.
b. Horner's syndrome.
c. Persisting pneumothorax.
d. Subcutaneous emphysema.
e. Haemothorax requiring drainage.

8 During a laparoscopic appendicectomy, you notice a sudden reduction in oxygen saturation associated with a low $EtCO_2$. Which one of the following would provide the earliest warning of gas embolism in this situation?

a. Use of a precordial Doppler.
b. Measurement of change in lung compliance.
c. Measurement of EtCO$_2$.
d. Use of pulse oximetry.
e. Use of an oesophageal stethoscope.

9

A 51-year-old male is admitted to the intensive care unit with severe sepsis secondary to community-acquired pneumonia. The patient is intubated, ventilated and commenced on inotropic support. The haematology results, 24 hours after admission show:

Hb 9.2g/dL, WCC 23.4 x 10^9/L, platelets 51 x 10^9/L, PT 23 seconds, fibrinogen 0.7g/L and raised D-dimers.

Clinical examination reveals a petechial rash all over his skin. From the list below, the most appropriate treatment of this patient's haematological condition would be:

a. Warfarin.
b. Antithrombin concentrate.
c. Transexamic acid.
d. Activated protein C.
e. Tissue factor prothrombin inhibitor (TFPI).

10

A 50-year-old man is scheduled for a laparotomy and biopsy of a mass originating from the appendix. A recent CT scan showed evidence of liver metastases. At anaesthetic pre-assessment, he describes a recent onset of diarrhoea and facial flushing. His GP has also recently diagnosed asthma and has prescribed inhalers. During the intra-operative period he suddenly becomes hypotensive as the mass is being manipulated by the surgeon. The most appropriate pharmacological management of this is:

a.   Intravenous ketanserin.
b.   Intravenous ephedrine 6mg.
c.   Intravenous metaraminol 1mg.
d.   Intravenous octreotide 10μg.
e.   Intravenous atracurium 10mg.

11

A 52-year-male has been suffering from pain in the right groin for the last 6 months. The pain started after hernia repair surgery and any identifiable reversible cause for this has been ruled out. Which of the following would be the most appropriate scale with which to assess his pain?

a.   Brief Pain Inventory.
b.   Visual Analogue Scale.
c.   Numeric Rating Scale.
d.   McGill Pain Questionnaire.
e.   Neuropathic Pain Scale.

12

A young male patient is admitted to a neurosurgical high dependency unit following a fall from a ladder. He is fully conscious and complains of pain over the posterior aspect of his neck. A CT scan of his cervical spine has revealed a non-displaced fracture at the level of C6-C7. Clinical examination reveals bilateral absent biceps reflexes and reduced sensation over the shoulders. About 8 hours later his SaO_2 decreases to 90% and blood gas analysis reveals a PaO_2 of 9kPa and $PaCO_2$ of 7.5kPa. The most likely cause of these abnormal blood gas results is:

a.   Diaphragmatic paralysis.
b.   Intercostal muscle paralysis.
c.   Respiratory centre depression.
d.   Pulmonary aspiration.
e.   Morphine overdose.

13 A 59-year-old male patient has had a hemi-arthroplasty of his right hip for a fractured neck of the femur. His past medical history includes heavy alcohol abuse and cirrhosis of the liver. During the intra-operative period the estimated blood loss was 1100ml and required two units of blood transfusion. During the immediate postoperative period his prothrombin time (PT) is noted to be 10 seconds above the control value, and the platelet count is 146 x 10^9/L. His haemoglobin is 9g/dL. From the list below the most appropriate therapeutic measure to correct the abnormal clotting is administration of:

a.   Packed red blood cells.
b.   Vitamin K.
c.   Fresh frozen plasma.
d.   Cryoprecipitate.
e.   Platelets.

14 A 25-year-old male is involved in a high speed road traffic accident. He has multiple injuries and is admitted to the intensive care unit after initial surgical stabilisation. On day two he deteriorates and requires intubation and ventilation for evolving ARDS. Later he requires haemofiltration due to acute renal failure and also requires inotropic support. Which of the following scoring systems will most accurately reflect the severity of his current clinical state and probability of mortality?

a.   Multiple Organ Dysfunction Score (MODS).
b.   Acute Physiology and Chronic Health Evaluation (APACHE) II score.
c.   Acute Physiology and Chronic Health Evaluation (APACHE) III score.
d.   Simplified Acute Physiology Score (SAPS).
e.   Injury Severity Score (ISS).

15 A 57-year-old male patient is scheduled for a nasal septoplasty. During the pre-operative assessment he is noted to be hypertensive. Further questioning reveals a history of headache, palpitations and sweating. Which of the following biochemical tests would be most sensitive in supporting the clinical diagnosis of pheochromocytoma?

a. Serum free metanephrine.
b. Urinary metanephrine.
c. Plasma catecholamines.
d. Urinary catecholamines.
e. Urinary vanillylmandelic acid.

16 A 37-year-old, ASA1 female patient with a mid-humeral fracture is scheduled for open reduction and internal fixation. She is very concerned about postoperative pain and has agreed to have a nerve block. Which one of the following nerve blocks is most likely to be the most successful in relieving her pain?

a. Supraclavicular brachial plexus block.
b. Interscalene brachial plexus block.
c. Cervical plexus block.
d. Axillary brachial plexus block.
e. Infraclavicular brachial plexus block.

17 A 75-year-old male patient with cardiovascular disease is being risk assessed prior to surgery. Which of the following independent factors carries the greatest risk?

a. Presence of a third heart sound.
b. Age >70 years.
c. Emergency procedure.
d. ECG showing atrial fibrillation.
e. Aortic surgery planned.

18 A 35-year-old female presents with weakness of the legs. An urgent MRI scan is organised which shows a disc prolapse at the L5/S1 vertebral level causing compression of the cauda equina. On neurological examination, which of the following clinical signs is likely to be present?

a. Extensor plantar response.
b. Brisk ankle jerks.
c. Weakness of hip flexion.
d. Peri-anal numbness.
e. Reduced knee jerks.

19 A 34-year-old woman presents to the emergency department following a road accident. She is conscious with a clear airway and adequate breathing. A CT scan shows a small splenic laceration with blood around the spleen. There is no blood in the peritoneum. No other injuries are identified. Following initial resuscitation with crystalloids her blood pressure stabilises at 110/70mm Hg and her pulse is 84/min. Her Hb is 12g/dL. What should be the next step in her management?

a. Blood transfusion.
b. Exploratory laparotomy.
c. Splenectomy.
d. Observation and monitoring.
e. Arterial embolisation.

20 A 4-year-old girl weighing 20kg was admitted to hospital for an elective tonsillectomy. During the procedure which was performed uneventfully, intravenous fluids were commenced using sodium chloride 0.18% with glucose 4% at a rate of 100ml/hour. She was discharged to the ward in the afternoon and intravenous fluids were continued at the same rate. The next day in the early morning she develops a generalised tonic-clonic seizure, which is treated with intravenous lorazepam. What should be done as a first step in her subsequent management?

a.   Measure urinary sodium level.
b.   Measure plasma electrolytes.
c.   Perform an urgent CT brain scan.
d.   Commence a phenytoin infusion.
e.   Check the plasma glucose.

21 A 14-year-old girl with sickle cell disease presents with severe chest and abdominal pain. For the last 2 years she has suffered from intermittent exacerbations every few weeks. During the acute exacerbations her pain always has been severe and is affecting her sleep and ability to attend school. Which one of the following would be the most suitable analgesic to manage her pain?

a.   Psychological counselling.
b.   Regular paracetamol.
c.   Regular diclofenac sodium.
d.   Regular morphine.
e.   Tunnelled thoracic epidural catheter.

22 A 33-year-old woman is admitted to the emergency department. She is known to have brittle asthma. She is admitted with an acute exacerbation; her peak flow is 40% of predicted and her pulse is 112 bpm. She has difficulty talking in sentences. Arterial blood gas shows a $PaCO_2$ of 3.9kPa. She is given oxygen, nebulised salbutamol and ipratropium bromide, and intravenous hydrocortisone. There is, however, no improvement. The next step in the subsequent management should be:

a.   Intravenous magnesium sulphate.
b.   Intravenous co-amoxiclav.
c.   Nebulised adrenaline.
d.   Arrange for non-invasive ventilation on intensive care.
e.   Intravenous aminophylline.

23 The results of pulmonary function tests performed on a patient complaining of exertional breathlessness are as follows: FEV1 2.4L (57% of predicted), FEV1/FVC ratio 0.8, DLCO reduced, DLCO/VA reduced. [DLCO = Diffusion lung capacity for carbon monoxide; VA = alveolar volume]. Which is the most likely diagnosis?

a. Pulmonary haemorrhage.
b. Emphysema.
c. Fibrosing alveolitis.
d. Asthma.
e. Pneumonectomy.

24 A 67-year-old gentleman without any previous medical problem was admitted with community-acquired pneumonia. His condition rapidly worsened over a few hours and he required mechanical ventilation. The most common causative agent likely to produce his community-acquired pneumonia is:

a. *Streptococcus pneumoniae.*
b. *Staphylococcus aureus.*
c. *Haemophilus influenzae.*
d. *Legionella pneumophilia.*
e. *Mycoplasma pneumoniae.*

25 A 3-year-old child has had an adenotonsillectomy. The operation itself was uneventful with minimal blood loss. Four hours after the procedure the child is found to be very irritable, pale, tachycardic and is spitting blood. Which of the following would be the next step in the management of this child?

a. Administration of I.V. morphine.
b. Suction of the mouth and pharynx.
c. Encourage the child to drink cold oral fluids.
d. The child should be returned to theatre and intubated immediately.
e. Administration of I.V. fluids and/or blood prior to induction of anaesthesia.

26 A 62-year-old female patient is scheduled for right hip hemi-arthroplasty. She has a history of angina, hypertension, and chronic obstructive airway disease. She has been on home oxygen 2L/minute, 4-6 hours per day, for the last 6 months. Which one of the following conditions would be an absolute contraindication to spinal anaesthesia in this patient?

a. Presence of urinary tract infection.
b. History of spinal bifida occulta.
c. Previous spinal decompression at the L5-S1 level.
d. History of multiple sclerosis.
e. Patient refusal.

27 A 35-year-old fit young woman is undergoing an internal fixation of her tibia under a general anaesthetic. While the surgeon is inserting the implant she develops sudden hypotension and her $EtCO_2$ shows a sudden drop from 5kPa to 2kPa. What is the most likely diagnosis?

a. Anaesthetic-induced myocardial depression.
b. Hypothermia.
c. Pulmonary embolism.
d. Massive haemorrhage.
e. Pneumothorax.

28 A 23-year-old primigravida was given a spinal anaesthetic for a Caesarean section after a prolonged labour and failure to progress. She had not used any labour analgesia. Prior to the block she had developed bilateral carpo-pedal spasm which resolved spontaneously soon after the subarachnoid block was established. The most likely diagnosis is:

a. Bupivacaine toxicity.
b. Hypocalcaemia.
c. Hypokalaemia.
d. Hypermagnesaemia.
e. Hypercapnia.

29 A young male had a splenectomy for blunt abdominal trauma 10 days ago. He now complains of upper abdominal pain worsened by deep breathing. His temperature is 38.4°C and he has decreased breath sounds over the left lung base. His respiratory rate is 20/minute and oxygen saturation is 99% on room air. His total white cell count is 15×10^9/L and a chest X-ray shows atelectasis in his lower lung field with a raised left hemi-diaphragm. Abdominal X-ray shows a non-specific gas pattern in the bowel and an air fluid level in the left upper quadrant. The most likely diagnosis is:

a. Diaphragmatic palsy.
b. Acute pancreatitis.
c. Sub-phrenic abscess.
d. Abdominal wound infection.
e. Hospital-acquired pneumonia.

30 A 2-year-old child is brought to the emergency department with acute onset of respiratory distress, cough and stridor. The chest appears hyperinflated on the right side with reduced movements and breath sounds. The child is irritable with an oxygen saturation of 90% on air and a heart rate of 120/minute. What is the most likely diagnosis?

a. Acute severe asthma.
b. Acute epiglottitis.
c. Aspiration pneumonia.
d. Foreign body aspiration.
e. Anaphylaxis.

Set 3 answers

1   Answer: E. Intravenous ondansetron 4mg.

Metoclopramide, prochlorperazine and droperidol can cause extrapyramidal side effects and worsen the symptoms of Parkinson's disease. Dexamethasone given to an awake patient can cause distressing perineal dysaesthesia. 5-HT3 receptor antagonists such as ondansetron are the most suitable for this patient. Cyclizine and domperidone (which do not cross the blood-brain barrier to any significant degree) are also safe to use in Parkinson's disease.

Further reading
1. Errington D, Severn A, Meara J. Parkinson's disease. *British Journal of Anaesthesia CEPD reviews* 2002; 2: 69-73.

†2   Answer: C. Transfuse 4 units of O-negative allogenic blood.

This patient is in haemorrhagic shock and the ST depression suggests myocardial hypoperfusion. She requires urgent blood transfusion. Although there is evidence that she is a Jehovah's Witness, there is no formal advance directive available and she is unable to express her wishes regarding blood transfusion due to coma. She must therefore be treated in her best interests with blood as this may be life-saving. Efforts can be made subsequently to establish her wishes. Some Jehovah's Witnesses may electively agree to a blood transfusion if it is clear that without this their life is in grave danger.

Cell salvage is acceptable to some Jehovah's Witnesses if the circuit is set up such that their blood is kept in continuity with their body. Intravenous iron can be useful in pre-operative optimisation or to treat anaemia but will not be of use in the emergency situation.

Further reading
1. Management of Anaesthesia for Jehovah's Witnesses, 2nd ed. Association of Anaesthetists of Great Britain and Ireland, 2005.

3   Answer: E. CPR, defibrillation, adrenaline, 20% Intralipid.

The cause of this woman's symptoms and cardiac arrest is likely to be due to intravascular injection of local anaesthetic (LA) leading to LA toxicity. The principles of managing cardiac arrest associated with LA toxicity are:

♦ To start cardiopulmonary resuscitation (CPR) using standard protocols.
♦ To manage arrhythmias using the same protocols, recognising that they may be very refractory to treatment.
♦ Prolonged resuscitation may be necessary; it may be appropriate to consider other options (cardiopulmonary bypass and continuing treatment with 20% Intralipid).

CPR should be continued throughout the treatment with the 20% Intralipid. After 4 minutes, preparations to perform an immediate Caesarean section should commence, aiming to deliver the foetus 5 minutes after cardiac arrest has occurred. A gravid uterus causes aortocaval compression which will only hamper resuscitation efforts; emptying the uterus affords the mother the best chance of survival.

Further reading
1. Guidelines for the management of severe local anaesthetic toxicity. Association of Anaesthetists of Great Britain and Ireland, 2007.
2. Cardiopulmoary resuscitation in the non-pregnant and pregnant woman. In: *Managing obstetric emergencies and trauma course manual*, 2nd ed. Grady K, Howell C, Cox C, Eds. Advanced Life Support Group 2007; Chapter 4; 21-9.

4 Answer: C. Intravenous immunoglobulin given over 5 days.

The two currently recognised disease-modifying modalities are intravenous immunoglobulin therapy and plasma exchange. Non-invasive ventilation is unlikely to be of benefit in a situation where clearance of secretions is a problem. Despite the anti-inflammatory actions of corticosteroids, there is no convincing evidence for the use of steroids. Pain killers, physiotherapy and mechanical ventilation will form a part of supportive management. Intravenous immunoglobulin therapy is easier to administer and has a similar efficacy to plasma exchange.

Further reading
1. Richards KJC, Cohen AT. Guillain-Barré syndrome. *British Journal of Anaesthesia CEPD Reviews* 2003; 3: 46-9.
2. Pritchard J. What's new in Guillain-Barré syndrome? *Postgrad Med J* 2008; 84: 532-8.

5 Answer: E. General anaesthesia with attenuation of the response to laryngoscopy and intubation.

The platelet count has decreased by one third in the last 12 hours, which is quite a precipitous fall. There is no test for platelet function, however, and clotting results are abnormally prolonged (INR and APTT are >1.5). The systolic blood pressure is adequately controlled. Given the clotting and platelet abnormalities, and the fact that the platelet count often drops in the 48 hours following delivery in haemolysis, elevated liver enzymes and low platelets (HELLP) syndrome, the best choice in this situation would be general anaesthesia, with attenuation of the response to laryngoscopy and intubation. This may be done by administering any of the following drugs prior to laryngoscopy:

- Alfentanil 20-30µg/kg.
- Magnesium sulphate 40mg/kg.
- Labetalol 0.25mg/kg.
- Esmolol 0.5mg/kg.
- Remifentanil 0.5µg/kg.

Further reading

1. HELLP syndrome. In: *Analgesia, anaesthesia and pregnancy – a practical guide*, 2nd ed, Yentis S, May A, Malhotra S, Eds. Cambridge, UK: Cambridge University Press, 2007; 80: 187-9.

2. The use of neuraxial anesthesia in parturients with thrombocytopenia: what is an adequate platelet count? In: *Evidence-based obstetric anesthesia*. Halpern SJ, Douglas M, Eds. London: BMJ Books, 2005.

6   Answer: B. Intrathecal opioid delivery via an implanted pump.

Drug toxicity and fear of drug toxicity are the leading causes of failure of cancer pain therapy. About 10% of cancer patients have refractory pain and require advanced techniques such as adjunct medications, nerve blocks, or an intrathecal implantable drug delivery system (IDDS). Systemic drugs relieve pain but often have serious side effects including sedation, confusion, constipation, or fatigue. These symptoms can be severe enough to limit the increment in the dose to an adequate level.

IDDSs deliver small doses of morphine directly into the cerebrospinal fluid (CSF), achieving pain relief with much smaller doses (1/300th of the oral dose). As the dose required is only a fraction of the oral or parenteral dose, side effects are significantly less. The IDDS consists of a small, battery-powered, programmable pump that is implanted under the skin of the abdomen and connected to a small intrathecal catheter.

In this patient a limiting factor in achieving satisfactory pain relief is the side effects of opioids, and this can be best addressed by an implantable IDDS. An epidural infusion would have a higher risk of infection and the dose required would be ten times higher than the intrathecal dose. All other mentioned options would reduce the dose and therefore not reduce the side effects.

Further reading

1. Smith TJ, *et al*. Randomized clinical trial of an implantable drug delivery system compared with comprehensive medical management for refractory cancer pain: impact on pain, drug-related toxicity, and survival. *Journal of Clinical Oncology* 2002; 20: 4040-9.

7 Answer: A. Compensatory sweating.

The indications for endoscopic thoracic sympathectomy include craniofacial hyperhydrosis, facial blushing, chronic regional pain syndromes, angina pectoris and congenital long QT syndrome. To treat palmar hydrosis the sympathetic chain is divided at the T2-4 level. The most common anaesthesia-related intra-operative complication is hypoxia and the most serious intra-operative surgical complication is injury to the subclavian vessels. The approximate incidence of postoperative complications is as follows:

- Compensatory sweating (back, trunk and thigh): 50-67%.
- Gustatory sweating: 28-47%.
- Persistent pneumothorax: 2-4%.
- Complete Horner's syndrome: 0.1.3%.
- Subcutaneous emphysema: 0-2%.
- Haemothorax requiring drainage: 0-2%.

Further reading
1. Martin A, Telford R. Anaesthesia for endoscopic thoracic sympathectomy. *British Journal of Anaesthesia CEACCP* 2009; 9: 52-5.

8 Answer A. Use of a precordial Doppler.

Venous gas embolism is a serious complication of laparoscopic surgery and is more common if excessive inflation pressures are used. Precordial Doppler ultrasound is the most sensitive method of detecting venous gas embolism. Unfortunately, it is not quantitative and does not differentiate between massive and physiologically insignificant embolism. Transoesophageal echocardiography allows determination of the volume of air, but is invasive and difficult to place. Practically, $EtCO_2$ is the most useful monitor as it is routinely available and sensitive. An oesophageal stethoscope may indicate the presence of a large embolus if a mill-wheel murmur is heard. There should be no change in pulmonary compliance when pulmonary embolism occurs.

Further reading

1. Webber S, Andrzejowski J, Francis G. Gas embolism in anaesthesia. *British Journal of Anaesthesia CEPD Reviews* 2002; 2: 53-7.

9   Answer: D. Activated protein C.

This patient meets the criteria for overt disseminated intravascular coagulation (DIC). The cornerstone of management is treatment of the underlying condition. Treatment with blood products (platelets, FFP, cryoprecipitate) should not be based solely on laboratory results and is better reserved for use in patients with evidence of bleeding.

Activated protein C should be considered in patients with severe sepsis and DIC. Manufacturer guidance advises against its use if the platelet count is $<30 \times 10^9/L$ or if there is a high risk of bleeding. Warfarin would promote bleeding and is not appropriate. In general, transexamic acid and antithrombin concentrate are not recommended. There is no evidence that TFPI increases survival rate.

Further reading

1. Levi M, Toh C, Thachil J, Watson H. Guidelines for the diagnosis and management of disseminated intravascular coagulation. *British Journal of Haematology* 2009; 145: 24-33.

10   Answer: D. Intravenous octreotide 10µg.

This patient has features indicative of carcinoid syndrome from a carcinoid tumour of the appendix. Flushing, diarrhoea and bronchospasm result from the systemic release of vasoactive amines. Mediators are metabolised in the liver via portal drainage; therefore, only when there are liver metastases will carcinoid syndrome result. Large swings in blood pressure can be seen when the tumour is manipulated. There is an exaggerated response to exogenous catecholamines. Histamine-releasing drugs should be avoided. Octreotide, a somatostatin analogue, prevents the release of vasoactive mediators from the tumour and is the best treatment of sudden severe hypotension. It suppresses the secretion of pituitary growth hormone (GH) and thyrotropin, and decreases the release of a variety of pancreatic islet cell hormones including insulin, glucagon, and vasoactive intestinal peptide (VIP).

Ketanserin is a 5-hydroxy-tryptamine (5-HT2) type 2 receptor antagonist, which also has some α-adrenoreceptor blocking effect. It has been used for the treatment of intra-operative hypertensive episodes in patients with carcinoid syndrome.

Further reading

1. Chinniah S, French J, Levy D. Serotonin and anaesthesia. *British Journal of Anaesthesia CEACCP* 2008; 8: 43-5.
2. Houghton K, Carter JA. Peri-operative management of carcinoid syndrome. *Anaesthesia* 1986; 41: 596-9.

11   Answer: D. McGill Pain Questionnaire.

This patient has post-surgical chronic pain. In the majority of cases, patients and relatives are fearful of the cause, prognosis, and treatment, and there may be an impact on the patient's work, family life and social life. Psychological factors can therefore play a larger part in the presentation. For these reasons, multidimensional assessment tools are more commonly used in the chronic than in the acute setting. Common multidimensional pain scales are the McGill Pain Questionnaire and the Brief Pain Inventory. These scales assess pain intensity as well as mood, behaviours, thoughts and beliefs, physiological effects and their interaction with each other. The McGill Pain Questionnaire is more comprehensive than the Brief Pain Inventory. The McGill Pain Questionnaire has been validated for the assessment of sensory, affective and evaluative aspects of chronic pain. It has also been used in research studies related to chronic pain. Visual analogue and numeric rating scales are designed to assess acute pain. The Neuropathic Pain Scale is designed to diagnose neuropathic pain and is not a multidimensional pain scale.

Further reading

1. Bruce J, Poobalan AS, Smith WC, Chambers WA. Quantitative assessment of chronic postsurgical pain using the McGill Pain Questionnaire. *Clin J Pain* 2004; 20: 70-5.

12   Answer: A. Diaphragmatic paralysis.

The blood gas result shows hypoxia and hypercapnia suggestive of ventilatory failure. This patient has a cervical spine injury below the level of the phrenic nerve and above the level of the cardiac sympathetic fibres. Although injury at this level can cause paralysis of intercostal and abdominal muscles, the patient is able to maintain adequate minute ventilation via the diaphragm and accessory muscles. Several hours later oedema of the spinal cord may result in ascending injury causing diaphragmatic paralysis.

Further reading

1.   Kang L, Tao-Chen L, Cheng-Loong L, *et al.* Delayed apnea in patients with mid- to lower cervical spinal cord injury. *Spine* 2000; 25: 1332-8.

13   Answer: C. Fresh frozen plasma.

As this patient has cirrhosis of the liver, he is likely to have deranged coagulation secondary to decreased synthesis of clotting factors in the liver, leading to an increased PT. An increase in the PT by only 2 seconds above the control values is likely to cause delayed coagulation. The haematological investigations reveal adequate levels of haemoglobin and platelets. Vitamin K administration helps in the synthesis of vitamin K dependent clotting factors, such as Factors II, VII, IX and X, but the effect is not immediate, taking at least 12-24 hours to work; it is also less effective in the presence of hepatic insufficiency.

The platelet count is within normal limits; therefore, platelet transfusion is not required for this patient. The low fibrinogen level can be corrected by transfusing cryoprecipitate. One adult dose of cryoprecipitate contains 3.2-4g of fibrinogen in a volume of 150-200ml. Cryoprecipitate also contains Factors VIII, XIII and von Willebrand Factor.

Further reading

1.   Feierman DE, Gaberielson GV. Liver disease. In: *Clinical cases in anaesthesia*, 3rd ed. Reed AP, Yudkowitz FS, Eds. Philadelphia, USA: Elsevier Churchill Livingstone, 2005; Case 35: 181-93.

14 Answer: A. Multiple Organ Dysfunction Score (MODS).

APACHE and SAPS are scores calculated on the first day of ICU admission only. In this case, these scores would have been relatively low, since on day 1 the patient was relatively well. Other scoring systems are repetitive and collect data sequentially throughout the duration of the ICU stay and, hence, would give worsening scores should the patient deteriorate, e.g. MODS, Sequential Organ Failure Assessment (SOFA) and Organ System Failure (OSF). ISS is an anatomical scoring system based on the location and types of injury following trauma.

Further reading
1. Bouch D, Thompson J. Severity scoring systems in the critically ill. *British Journal of Anaesthesia CEACCP* 2008; 8: 181-5.

15 Answer: A. Serum free metanephrine.

Plasma free metanephrines provide the best test for the diagnosis of pheochromocytoma. Sensitivities of plasma free metanephrines is 99% and urinary fractionated metanephrines (97%) are higher than those for plasma catecholamines (84%) and urinary catecholamines (86%). Specificity is highest for urinary vanillylmandelic acid (95%) and urinary total metanephrines (93%).

Further reading
1. Lenders JW, Pacak K, *et al.* Biochemical diagnosis of phaeochromocytoma: which test is best? *JAMA* 2002; 287: 1427-34.

16 Answer: A. Supraclavicular brachial plexus block.

The brachial plexus is formed by C5, C6, C7, C8, and T1 nerve roots. In the supraclavicular region, the brachial plexus is most compact as at this level roots join to form the trunks. Blockade at this level has the greatest likelihood of blocking all the branches of the plexus and has a high success rate. The apex of the lung is just medial and posterior to the brachial plexus at this level and there is a relatively high risk of pneumothorax occurring. To minimize this risk, the needle should not be directed too medially.

The interscalene approach is also indicated for shoulder surgery. It is the most proximal approach to the brachial plexus, a paravertebral approach at the level of the cervical roots in the neck. The areas supplied by C8 and T1 nerve roots may prove difficult to block and this approach is therefore less suitable for surgery involving the area supplied by the ulnar nerve.

Further reading

1. Neal JM, *et al.* Brachial plexus anaesthesia: essentials of our current understanding. *Reg Anesth Pain Med* 2002; 27: 402-28.
2. Pinnock CA, Fischer HBJ, Jones RP. *Peripheral nerve blockade.* Edinburgh: Churchill Livingstone, 1996.

17   Answer: A. Presence of a third heart sound.

The Goldman Risk Index uses nine independent risk factors which are evaluated on a point scale:

- Third heart sound (S3): 11 (as this is a sign of left ventricular dysfunction).
- Elevated jugular venous pressure: 11.
- Myocardial infarction in the past 6 months: 10.
- ECG: premature atrial contractions or any rhythm other than sinus: 7.
- ECG shows >5 premature ventricular contractions per minute: 7.
- Age >70 years: 5.
- Emergency procedure: 4.
- Intra-thoracic, intra-abdominal or aortic surgery: 3.
- Poor general status, metabolic or bedridden: 3.

Patients with scores >25 have a 56% incidence of death, and a 22% incidence of severe cardiovascular complications.

Patients with scores <25 but >6 have a 4% incidence of death, and a 17% incidence of severe cardiovascular complications.

Patients with scores <6 have a 0.2% incidence of death, and a 0.7% incidence of severe cardiovascular complications.

Further reading
1. Goldman L, Caldera DL, Nussbaum SR, *et al.* Multifactorial index of cardiac risk in noncardiac surgical procedures. *N Engl J Med* 1977; 297: 845-50.

18 Answer: D. Peri-anal numbness.

Cauda equina syndrome causes lower motor neurone signs in the lower limbs, the precise features of which depend upon on the level of compression. Lower motor neurone signs include: muscle wasting, fasciculations, flaccid paralysis, absent/reduced reflexes and a flexor plantar response. Compression of L5, S1 nerve roots can cause peri-anal numbness (saddle anaesthesia), sensory loss along the lateral aspect of the foot, an absent ankle jerk and loss of bowel and bladder function. Hip flexion is a function of L2 and L3 nerve roots and the knee jerk involves L3 and L4 nerve roots.

Further reading
1. Small SA, Perron AD, Brady WJ. Orthopedic pitfalls: cauda equina syndrome. *American Journal of Emergency Medicine* 2005; 23: 159-63.

19 Answer: D. Observation and monitoring.

Isolated solid organ injury in a haemodynamically normal patient can often be managed conservatively. Such patients must be admitted to hospital for careful observation. Evaluation by a surgeon is essential. Concomitant hollow viscus injury occurs in less than 5% of patients initially thought to have isolated solid organ injuries.

Further reading
1. Abdominal trauma. In: *ATLS manual,* 7th ed., 2004: 141.

20 Answer: B. Measure plasma electrolytes.

This child has been given hypotonic fluid as a maintenance regime and this has been administered at a high rate for a long period of time. The child weighs 20kg, and using the '4-2-1' rule she should have received fluid at a rate of 60ml/hr. Severe hyponatraemia is the most likely explanation for the seizure and plasma levels need to be urgently measured. Hypoglycaemia is unlikely given the glucose-containing fluid being infused.

Hyponatraemia (serum Na <135mmol/l) may occur following surgery with any fluid regime, particularly if hypotonic maintenance fluids are given. The early signs are non-specific and often the first presenting feature is a seizure, or even respiratory arrest. Children with hyponatraemic encephalopathy should be managed as a medical emergency and transferred to a paediatric intensive care unit. Hyponatraemic seizures respond poorly to anticonvulsants and initial management is to give an infusion of 3% sodium chloride.

Further reading
1. Association of Paediatric Anaesthetists of Great Britain and Ireland. APA consensus guideline on perioperative fluid management in children. London: Association of Paediatric Anaesthetists of Great Britain and Ireland, 2007.

21 Answer: D. Regular morphine.

Pain is the most frequent problem experienced by patients with sickle cell disease. The frequency and severity of painful episodes are highly variable among patients. Painful episodes may start in the first year of life and continue thereafter. The episodes last from hours to weeks followed by a return to baseline. Dehydration, infection, stress, fatigue, menstruation and cold can precipitate painful episodes. Medication is one of the mainstays of treatment during the acute episode. Medication includes paracetamol, non-steroidal anti-inflammatory drugs (NSAIDs), opioids, adjuvants such as tricyclic antidepressants, and invasive approaches such as epidural analgesia. Painful crises are treated symptomatically with analgesics. The milder crises can be managed using NSAIDs and paracetamol, but most patients with severe crises such as this will require opioids.

NSAIDs are often considered benign and preferable to opioids. However, particular risks such as blood loss from occult gastritis and analgesic nephropathy are possible from long-term use. In this patient the exacerbations are frequent and severe, and use of regular morphine would be indicated in order to manage the pain.

Further reading
1. Ballas SK. Current issues in sickle cell pain and its management. Hematology American Society of Education program book, 2007: 97-105.

22   Answer: A. Intravenous magnesium sulphate.

The severity of exacerbations of asthma can be assessed using the criteria of the British Thoracic Society. A severe exacerbation can be defined as having any one of the following features:

-   PEFR 33-50% best or predicted.
-   Heart rate >110 bpm or respiratory rate >25.
-   Inability to complete sentences in one breath.

Pulse oximetry, arterial blood gases and chest X-ray are useful investigations. Oxygen, nebulised β2-agonists and ipratropium bromide, and steroids should be administered.

If there is a poor initial response to inhaled bronchodilators, a single dose of magnesium sulphate should be given (1.2-2g intravenous infusion over 20 minutes). Routine prescription of antibiotics for acute asthma is not indicated.

The role of intravenous aminophylline in acute asthma is now less clear. Patients with a poor response to initial therapy may gain benefit from treatment. Such patients are probably rare and could not be identified in a meta-analysis of trials. Side effects of aminophylline include arrhythmias and vomiting.

Hypercapnic respiratory failure developing during an acute asthmatic episode is an indication for urgent ICU admission. It is unlikely that non-invasive ventilation (NIV) would replace intubation in these very unstable patients, but it has been suggested that treatment is safe and effective.

Further reading

1. Scottish Intercollegiate Guidelines Network: British guideline on the management of asthma (SIGN guideline 101). Edinburgh: SIGN, 2009. (http://www.sign.ac.uk/pdf/sign101.pdf).

23 Answer: C. Fibrosing alveolitis.

Spirometry is useful in distinguishing obstructive lung disease from restrictive lung disease. A low FEV1 with a normal/raised FEV1/FVC is suggestive of restrictive lung disease. Lung volume measurements showing reduced total lung capacity (TLC) are the hallmark of restrictive disease.

In obstructive lung disease (e.g. COPD, asthma), both FEV1 and the FEV1/FVC ratio are reduced. There may be an increase in residual volume (RV) and TLC. This is particularly marked in emphysema.

DLCO, also known as the transfer factor of the lung for carbon monoxide, is a measure of the diffusing capacity from alveolar gas to the red blood cells in the pulmonary circulation. It is helpful in evaluating the presence of possible parenchymal lung disease when spirometry and/or lung volume determinations suggest a reduced vital capacity, RV, and/or TLC. Because the DLCO is directly proportional to VA, non-pulmonary processes that reduce the TLC cause reductions in the DLCO. If VA can be assessed accurately, these reductions produce a normal or elevated DL/VA ratio, e.g. lung resection, thoracic cage abnormalities. A reduced DLCO and a reduced DL/VA ratio suggest a true interstitial disease such as pulmonary fibrosis or pulmonary vascular disease.

Further reading

1. Plummer AL. The carbon monoxide diffusing capacity. *Chest* 2008; 134: 663-7.

24 Answer: A. *Streptococcus pneumoniae.*

Although all of the above mentioned agents can produce community-acquired pneumonia, the most common agent causing it is *Streptococcus pneumoniae.* Patients suffering from severe community-acquired pneumonia are more likely to suffer secondary infections by other organisms, for example, *S. aureus, P. aeruginosa* and other gram-negative bacilli.

Further reading
1. Lim WS, *et al.* BTS guidelines for the management of community-acquired pneumonia in adults: update 2009. *Thorax* 2009; 64 (Suppl III): iii1-55

25 Answer: E. Administration of I.V. fluids and/or blood prior to induction of anaesthesia.

This child is showing signs of significant post-tonsillectomy haemorrhage. The usual cause of blood loss is venous or capillary ooze from the tonsillar bed and it is difficult to measure, as it occurs over several hours and is partly swallowed. Excessive blood loss may lead to the child spitting blood. In these cases, the child is likely to be seriously hypovolaemic, anaemic and potentially difficult to intubate because of poor visualization of the larynx. Pre-operative resuscitation (guided by trends in monitoring) is essential, as induction of anaesthesia in a hypovolaemic child can precipitate cardiovascular collapse. Anaesthesia is induced once the child is haemodynamically stable. Preoxygenation and rapid sequence induction with a slight head-down positioning of the patient ensures rapid control of the airway and protection from pulmonary aspiration.

Further reading
1. Ravi R, Howell T. Anaesthesia for paediatric ear, nose, and throat surgery. *British Journal of Anaesthesia CEACCP* 2007; 7: 33-7.

26 Answer: E. Patient refusal.

If patients have the capacity to make decisions for themselves, patient refusal is an absolute contraindication to any procedure. The basic principles of consent in a patient with capacity are:

- The doctor uses specialist knowledge and experience to make a clinical judgement, and taking the patient's views and understanding of their condition, identifies which investigations or treatments are likely to result in overall benefit for the patient. The doctor explains the options to the patient, setting out the potential benefits, risks, burdens and side effects of each option, including the option of having no treatment. The doctor may recommend a particular option which they believe to be best for the patient, but they must not put undue pressure on the patient to accept their advice.
- The patient weighs up the potential benefits and risks of the various options as well as any non-clinical issues that are relevant to them, then decides whether to accept any of the options and, if so, which one. They also have the right to accept or refuse an option for a reason that may seem irrational to the doctor or for no reason at all.

In all of the other mentioned conditions, spinal anaesthesia can be performed with care. Severe coagulopathy and severe sepsis are also absolute contraindications to neuraxial anaesthesia.

Further reading

1. General Medical Council. Consent guidance: patients and doctors making decisions together, 2008. (http://www.gmc-uk.org/guidance /ethical_guidance/consent_guidance_index.asp).
2. O'Rourke N, Khan K, Hepner DL. Contraindications to neuraxial anaesthesia. In: *Spinal and epidural anesthesia*. Wong CA, Ed. USA: McGraw Hill Medical, 2007; Chapter 5: 127-50.

27 Answer: C. Pulmonary embolism.

The increased intra-medullary pressure during nailing of long bones can lead to fat embolism. Apart from haemodynamic changes there may be hypoxia, pulmonary oedema, development of a coagulation disorder and CNS changes leading to convulsions or coma if the patient is awake. The sudden drop in EtCO$_2$ in this case is due to an increase in the alveolar dead space.

Further reading
1. Wiersema UF. Chest Injuries. In: *Oh's intensive care manual*, 6th ed. Bersten A, Soni N, Eds. Elsevier, 2009: 800.

28   Answer: B. Hypocalcaemia.

Without analgesia, a labouring woman can demonstrate a very high hyperventilatory response, with marked hypocapnia (PaCO$_2$ as low as 2kPa). This can lead to an acute reduction in ionised calcium leading to these symptoms.

Further reading
1. Ray N, Camann W. Hyperventilation-induced tetany associated with epidural analgesia for labour. *International Journal of Obstetric Anaesthesia* 2005; 14: 74-6.

29   Answer: C. Sub-phrenic abscess.

This patient shows signs of sepsis with symptoms mainly localizing to the left upper abdomen. A sub-phrenic abscess usually produces elevation of the left hemi-diaphragm, pleural effusion and basal atelectasis. The abscess can be confirmed by a CT scan or ultrasound. Unilateral diaphragmatic palsy can produce a raised hemi-diaphragm, seen on the chest X-ray. Acute pancreatitis can present with epigastric pain, pyrexia and shock. Usually there is a history of alcohol abuse, dyspepsia or biliary colic. In this patient, as there is a history of recent trauma and abdominal surgery, a sub-phrenic abscess is the most likely diagnosis. The clinical features are also suggestive of a chest infection, but the abdominal X-ray showing air fluid level suggests intra-abdominal pathology.

Further reading

1. Padley S. Imaging the chest. In: *Oh's intensive care manual*, 6th ed. Bersten A, Soni N, Eds. Elsevier, 2009: 466.

30   Answer: D. Foreign body aspiration.

Aspiration of a foreign body, commonly food, has a peak incidence at 1-2 years of age. A sudden onset of coughing, gagging, and choking suggest foreign body aspiration and may necessitate basic life support manoeuvres for the choking child. Partial obstruction of a lower airway may cause air trapping behind the foreign body (ball and valve effect) with pneumothorax, surgical emphysema, and pneumo-mediastinum a possibility. In this situation, the usual inspiratory chest X-ray can appear normal; an expiratory film, however, if it can be obtained, may reveal air trapping.

Further reading

1. Maloney E, Meakin GH. Acute stridor in children. *British Journal of Anaesthesia CEACCP* 2007; 183-6.
2. Warshawsky ME. Foreign body aspiration. (http://emedicine. medscape.com/article/298940-overview).

Set 4 questions

1   A 60-year-old female patient is admitted to the neurosurgical unit with a subarachnoid haemorrhage secondary to a ruptured intracranial aneurysm. Which of the following is the most serious complication that could occur during the subsequent 3 days?

a.   Re-bleeding.
b.   Cerebral vasospasm.
c.   Hypertension.
d.   Hydrocephalus.
e.   Pulmonary oedema.

2   A 70-year-old male patient is undergoing an oesophagectomy via a thoraco-abdominal approach requiring one-lung ventilation. Which of the following pathophysiological changes is least likely to occur during one-lung ventilation?

a.   Hypercarbia.
b.   Hypoxia.
c.   Intrapulmonary shunt.
d.   Hypoxic pulmonary vasoconstriction.
e.   Ventilation perfusion mismatch.

3 A 67-year-old male patient has been anaesthetised with total intravenous anaesthesia using propofol and remifentanil for an inguinal hernia repair. About 10 minutes after induction his blood pressure falls to 80/50mmHg and heart rate to 42 per minute. The immediate treatment should be:

a. Intravenous ephedrine.
b. Intravenous metaraminol.
c. Intravenous phenylephrine.
d. Reducing the dose of propofol.
e. I.V. infusion of 1L of normal saline.

4 A 72-year-old man underwent abdominopelvic resection of a carcinoma of the rectum. On the third postoperative day he developed right-sided chest pain with no new ST-T changes on the ECG. Clinical examination revealed a temperature of 37.6°C, SpO_2 of 88% (on 15L/min of oxygen via a non-rebreathing mask), tachypnoea, tachycardia with a pulse rate of 130 per minute and a BP of 128/66mm Hg. Auscultation of the chest was unremarkable and the chest X-ray was normal. An arterial blood gas while on 15L/min oxygen revealed the following: pH 7.46kPa, $PaCO_2$ 4.8kPa, PaO_2 7.1kPa, lactate 1.2mmol/L and HCO_3^- 20mmol/L. The most likely diagnosis is:

a. Postoperative pneumonia.
b. Bibasal atelectasis.
c. Severe sepsis.
d. Acute coronary syndrome.
e. Pulmonary embolism.

5 A 36-year-old female patient presents for emergency appendicectomy. Two weeks ago she underwent scleral buckle repair of a spontaneous retinal detachment of the right eye. The most important precaution to be taken during the anaesthetic for her appendicectomy to avoid damage to her eye is:

a. Avoiding rapid sequence induction.
b. Avoiding nitrous oxide.
c. Avoiding hypercarbia.
d. Maintaining normocarbia.
e. Avoiding hypotension.

6 A patient is undergoing a percutaneous, X-ray-guided coeliac plexus block for the management of pain due to chronic pancreatitis. What position should the needle tip be in to provide the most effective block?

a. Anterior to the pancreas.
b. Anterior to the aorta.
c. Lateral to the inferior vena cava.
d. Posterior to the aorta.
e. Antero-lateral to the L1 vertebral body.

7 A 50-year-old patient is undergoing a posterior fossa craniotomy in the sitting position. Anaesthesia and surgery proceed uneventfully until approximately 2 hours into the procedure, when a sudden decrease in $EtCO_2$, a slight increase in heart rate and a reduction in blood pressure are noticed. Venous air embolism is suspected. The most sensitive clinical monitor in this situation would be:

a. Transoesophageal Doppler.
b. Precordial stethoscope.
c. $EtCO_2$ monitor.
d. Pulse oximeter.
e. PA catheter.

8 A young ASA1 patient underwent an elective abdominal hysterectomy under general anaesthesia with endotracheal intubation. She had no history of acid reflux. Soon after extubation, the patient developed severe laryngospasm which responded to intravenous propofol and CPAP via a face mask. Despite having a clear upper airway, she

remained breathless with an oxygen saturation of 90% whilst breathing 100% oxygen via a face mask. The oxygenation improved over a period of 2 hours following the use of CPAP and diuretic treatment. The most likely diagnosis in this patient is:

a. Aspiration pneumonia.
b. Negative pressure pulmonary oedema.
c. Bronchial asthma.
d. Fluid overload.
e. Congestive cardiac failure.

9 A 33-year-old woman is brought to the emergency department with a suspected drug overdose. She is drowsy, with tachycardia, hypotension and dilated pupils. Blood gases reveal a metabolic acidosis. The ECG shows sinus tachycardia with a QRS duration of 140ms. From the following which drug is she most likely to have taken as an overdose?

a. Phenytoin.
b. Fluoxetine.
c. Ethylene glycol.
d. Amitryptiline.
e. Amphetamine.

10 A 60-year-old male patient has undergone repair of a thoraco-abdominal aortic aneurysm. On the third postoperative day, 8 hours following discontinuation of epidural analgesia, he complains of an inability to move the lower limbs. Clinical examination reveals paraplegia with absence of cold and pain sensation with preserved sensation of deep touch, vibration and proprioception. The most likely diagnosis is:

a. Transverse myelitis.
b. Epidural haematoma.
c. Epidural abscess.
d. Anterior spinal artery syndrome. ←
e. Posterior spinal artery syndrome.

11 A 50-year-old male patient is scheduled for amputation of his great toe under regional anaesthesia. Which one of the following groups of nerves needs to be blocked to provide effective anaesthesia?

a. Deep peroneal and superficial nerves.
b. Deep peroneal nerve.
c. Deep peroneal and saphenous nerves.
d. Deep peroneal and superficial peroneal, and posterior tibial nerves.
e. Superficial peroneal and posterior tibial nerves.

12 A 35-year-old lady with a history of two previous Caesarean sections is undergoing a third Caesarean section under spinal anaesthesia. After the baby is delivered she develops an ongoing postpartum haemorrhage due to uterine atony. She has already received five units of oxytocin I.V. and 500µg ergometrine I.M. An oxytocin infusion (40 units in 500ml) has been commenced at a rate of 125ml/hour. What would be the next choice of drug for pharmacological management of her atonic PPH?

a. I.M. carboprost 250µg repeated at 15-minute intervals if necessary.
b. Intra-myometrial injection of carboprost 250µg.
c. A further 10 units of I.V. oxytocin as a bolus.
d. A repeat dose of I.V. ergometrine 500µg.
e. Rectal misoprostol 400µg.

13 A young female patient with isolated moderate mitral regurgitation is scheduled for a laparotomy and removal of an ovarian tumour. Which of the following statements would describe the best peri-operative haemodynamic goals for this patient?

a. Use of spinal anaesthesia to reduce the SVR.
b. Maintenance of normal SVR with a slow heart rate in order to maintain a favourable myocardial oxygen demand-supply ratio.

c. Use of an inhalational anaesthetic in preference to intravenous agents in order to achieve pulmonary vasodilation.
d. Maintenance of normal SVR using an I.V. infusion of metaraminol if required.
e. Maintenance of a normal to high heart rate avoiding sudden bradycardia, and maintenance of a normal to low SVR.

14 A 65-year-old female patient with rheumatoid arthritis presents to the emergency department with chest pain, shortness of breath and a low-grade fever of 3 days' duration. Her medications include prednisolone and methotrexate. Auscultation of the chest reveals a pericardial rub. The 12-lead ECG shows diffuse ST elevation with a heart rate of 110 per minute. The most likely diagnosis is:

a. Congestive cardiac failure.
b. Pericardial effusion.
c. Cardiac tamponade.
d. Myocardial infarction.
e. Pericarditis.

15 A 52-year-old woman presents for a right hemi-arthroplasty following a fall and sustaining a fractured neck of the femur. She has a history of alcoholic liver disease. On clinical examination she is fully conscious and orientated in time and place. She is jaundiced, but has no signs of hepatic encephalopathy, and there is no ascites. Biochemistry investigations reveal an increased prothrombin time (5 seconds above the control), the serum bilirubin is 3mg/dL and the serum albumin is 32g/L. Which of the following statements describe most accurately her likely peri-operative mortality?

a. She has a low operative mortality.
b. Her operative mortality is about 25%.
c. Her operative mortality is less than 5%.
d. According to modified Child's criteria she has a total score of 5.
e. According to modified Child's criteria she has a total score of 10.

16 A 32-year-old male is admitted to the high dependency unit for observation following a road traffic accident. He has sustained fractures of the 3rd, 4th, and 5th ribs on the right side with associated pain. You want to perform an intercostal nerve block for the management of the pain. At which site should the block be performed?

a.   Anterior axillary line.
b.   Mid-axillary line.
c.   Posterior axillary line.
d.   Posterior angle of the rib.
e.   At the fracture site.

17 A 23-year-old previously fit male presents with increasing dyspnoea. He has undergone cardiac catheterisation and the results of this investigation are shown in Table 1.

Table 1. Results of cardiac catheterisation.							
Cardiac chamber	**RA**	**RV**	**PA**	**PA wedge**	**LA**	**LV**	**Aorta**
Pressure in mmHg	4	12	45	9	5	110/8	110/70

The most likely diagnosis in this patient is:

a.   Mitral stenosis.
b.   Mitral incompetence.
c.   Aortic stenosis.
d.   Idiopathic pulmonary hypertension.
e.   Aortic incompetence.

18 A 27-year-old primigravida who is 37 weeks' pregnant is admitted to the labour ward with symptoms of headache, blurring of vision and confusion. On examination she has a blood pressure of 190/110mm Hg with increased reflexes, clonus and 3+ of protein in the urine. Which one of the following is the most appropriate treatment?

a. Oral labetalol.
b. Immediate delivery.
c. Hydralazine and magnesium.
d. Continue close monitoring and initiate treatment if she deteriorates.
e. Oral methyldopa.

19 A middle-aged female patient has been admitted to the intensive care unit with an acute exacerbation of asthma. On admission she was hypoxic, hypercarbic and tachycardic with a reduced level of consciousness. She was therefore sedated and ventilated manually initially in order to improve her oxygenation. Over a period of a few minutes she became hypotensive and more tachycardic and hypoxic. The most likely cause for her deterioration following ventilation was:

a. Pneumonia.
b. Tension pneumothorax.
c. Sepsis.
d. Hypovolaemia.
e. Myocardial infarction.

20 A 35-year-old female patient has had a laparoscopic cholecystectomy performed under general anaesthesia. The airway was secured using an orotracheal tube. A nasogastric tube was inserted using Magill forceps under direct vision with the aid of a laryngoscope to decompress the stomach. At the end of the procedure the trachea was extubated following blind suction using a Yankauer sucker. On transfer to the recovery room she developed breathing difficulties, and her oxygen saturation decreased to 94% despite 40% supplemental oxygen. No improvement was noted

despite administration of nebulised epinephrine. Examination of the oropharynx revealed a large oedematous uvula. Which of the following would be the most effective next step in her management?

a.   Intravenous dexamethasone.
b.   Intravenous hydrocortisone.
c.   Saline nebulisation.
d.   CPAP by face mask.
e.   Sedation and tracheal intubation.

21 In which of the following conditions is chronic post-surgical pain most commonly seen?

a.   Cholecystectomy.
b.   Mastectomy.
c.   Amputation of limb.
d.   Thoracotomy.
e.   Hernia repair.

 22 A 76-year-old female underwent a hemi-arthroplasty under general anaesthesia. A lumbar plexus block was performed at induction to provide postoperative analgesia. During the intra-operative period she required a transfusion of 2 units of blood. In the recovery room she is confused, disorientated and agitated. Her pain appears to be adequately controlled. Her vital parameters in recovery are shown in Table 2. 40% oxygen has been administered via a face mask.

Table 2. Vital parameters in recovery.				
Pulse rate	BP	Respiratory rate	SpO$_2$	Temperature
86 bpm	164/88 mmHg	14 bpm	97%	36.9°C

Despite all measures it is difficult to control her agitation. The following is the most appropriate pharmacological treatment in this patient:

a.   Midazolam 2mg I.V.
b.   Haloperidol 0.5-1mg I.V.
c.   Titrated doses of diazepam.
d.   Ketamine 0.25mg/kg I.V.
e.   Propofol 50-100mg I.V.

23 A 24-year-old woman who has been in prolonged labour is undergoing an emergency Caesarean section for failure to progress. During the procedure she loses about 3L of blood. The most likely cause for this massive haemorrhage is:

a.   Trauma to the cervix and birth canal.
b.   Primary coagulopathy.
c.   Disseminated intravascular coagulopathy.
d.   Uterine atony.
e.   Retained products of conception.

24 A 68-year-old man is admitted to the intensive care unit with severe sepsis and acute renal failure. He is commenced on continuous veno-venous haemodiafiltration, using unfractionated heparin as an anticoagulant. Sometime later it is noted that his platelet count has fallen. His platelet count on admission to the unit was 386 x 10^9/L. Which of the following laboratory results makes a diagnosis of type 2 heparin-induced thrombocytopaenia (HIT) more likely?

a.   Platelet count of 102 x 10^9/L 6 days after starting heparin.
b.   Lowest platelet count of 12 x 10^9/L during the treatment period.
c.   Detection of PF4-heparin IgA antibodies.
d.   Platelet count of 297 x 10^9/L 2 days after stopping heparin administration.
e.   Fibrinogen level of 0.6g/L.

25 A middle-aged male patient with a history of alcohol abuse presents to the accident and emergency department with a bout of prolonged vomiting followed by a massive haematemesis. Clinical examination reveals tachycardia, tachypnoea and hypotension. His body temperature is normal. Stool examination is negative for occult blood. The most likely diagnosis is:

a. Peptic ulcer.
b. Oesophageal stricture.
c. Reflux oesophagitis.
d. Hiatus hernia.
e. Mallory-Weiss syndrome.

26 A 52-year-old patient is known to have ischaemic heart disease, and has a permanent pacemaker. He is on various cardiac medications and had a CABG a year ago. He continues to suffer from chest pain and has been diagnosed with refractory angina. He also suffers from obstructive sleep apnoea and uses CPAP during the night. Which of the following would be the most appropriate treatment to manage his chest pain?

a. TENS therapy.
b. Stellate ganglion block.
c. Regular NSAIDs.
d. Regular diamorphine.
e. Fentanyl patch.

27 A 30-year-old male patient underwent open reduction and internal fixation of a fracture of the neck of the right humerus. Three weeks later he presents with an inability to lift the right arm. On examination there is reduced sensation over the lower part of the right deltoid region. Which of the following nerves are likely to have been injured thus causing his symptoms?

a. The axillary nerve.
b. The median nerve.
c. The suprascapular nerve.
d. The musculocutaneous nerve.
e. The radial nerve.

28 A 70-year-old man presents in the emergency department with a history of sudden onset of severe back ache. His past medical history includes hypertension, hypercholesterolaemia and a 5cm abdominal aortic aneurysm diagnosed 3 years before. On clinical examination his radial pulse is weak with a rate of 115 per minute; his blood pressure is 84/60mm Hg. There is a pulsatile mass in the epigastrium. The most likely diagnosis is:

a. Acute cholecystitis.
b. Acute gastritis.
c. Acute pancreatitis.
d. Ruptured abdominal aortic aneurysm.
e. Acute lumbar disc prolapse.

29 A 60-year-old male patient developed laryngospasm on the first postoperative day following a total thyroidectomy for carcinoma of the thyroid. Which of the following investigations is likely to be the most useful in the further management of this patient?

a. Serum magnesium.
b. Nasendoscopy to assess the vocal cord function.
c. Serum calcium.
d. Serum TSH.
e. Electrocardiogram.

30 A 40-year-old male patient underwent neck dissection and excision of a tumour on the floor of the mouth. Two weeks later he complains of a loss of taste sensation. Which one of the following nerves is likely to be injured during this surgery?

a. Inferior alveolar nerve.
b. Lingual nerve.
c. Glossopharyngeal nerve.
d. Buccal nerve.
e. Hypoglossal nerve.

Set 4 answers

1   Answer: A. Re-bleeding.

Although cerebral vasospasm is the most common problem, the most serious complication of subarachnoid haemorrhage (SAH) is re-bleeding; the occurrence is about 15% during the first week. The management of cerebral vasospasm consists of nimodipine and triple H therapy (induced hypertension, hypervolaemia and haemodilution). SAH is also frequently associated with systemic and pulmonary hypertension, cardiac arrhythmias and neurogenic pulmonary oedema. Other complications include hydrocephalus and electrolyte disturbances. Hyponatraemia develops as a result of either cerebral salt wasting syndrome or the syndrome of inappropriate ADH secretion.

Further reading
1. Solenski NJ, Haley E, *et al*. Medical complications of aneurysmal subarachnoid hemorrhage: a report of the multicenter, cooperative aneurysm study. *Critical Care Medicine* 1995; 23: 1007-17.
2. Priebe H-J. Aneurysmal subarachnoid haemorrhage and the anaesthetist. *British Journal of Anaesthesia* 2007; 99: 102-18.

2   Answer: A. Hypercarbia.

Patients undergoing oesophagectomy are positioned in the lateral decubitus position. During surgery, once the non-dependent lung is collapsed, ventilation to that lung is eliminated. The blood passing through the collapsed non-dependent lung does not take part in gas exchange, possibly resulting in hypoxia. CO_2 exchange is not affected to the same extent as oxygenation. The blood passing through the collapsed, non-ventilated lung contributes to the ventilation perfusion mismatch and shunt.

Further reading
1. Neustin SM, Eisenkraft JB. One-lung anesthesia. In: *Clinical cases in anaesthesia*, 3rd ed. Reed AP, Yudkowitz FS, Eds. Philadelphia, USA: Elsevier Churchill Livingstone, 2005; Case 15: 73-84.

3 Answer: A. Intravenous ephedrine.

This patient has bradycardia with hypotension, most likely caused by remifentanil. This should best respond to intravenous ephedrine and reducing the dose of remifentanil. Speed of injection is an important factor for bradycardia with remifentanil, commonly seen with administration of a bolus dose. The incidence of bradycardia may be minimized by slow administration. It is generally accepted that the bradycardia is vagally mediated and bilateral vagotomy has been shown to abolish this effect.

Ephedrine acts both directly by causing release of noradrenaline from the sympathetic nerve terminals, and indirectly by stimulation of α and β adrenoreceptors. It has positive chronotropic and inotropic effects on the heart.

Metaraminol also has both direct and indirect sympathomimetic effects. It stimulates both α and β adrenoreceptors, but α effects predominate causing an increase in systemic vascular resistance. It increases both systolic and diastolic blood pressure, and a reflex bradycardia occurs which may further decrease the heart rate in this patient.

Phenylephrine is a selective $\alpha 1$ agonist, which has no chronotropic effect. It can be used in situations where peripheral vasoconstriction is needed and cardiac output is adequate, as in hypotension that may accompany spinal anaesthesia.

Further reading
1. DeSouza G, Lewis MC, TerRiet MF. Severe bradycardia after remifentanil. *Anesthesiology* 1997; 87: 1019-20.

4   Answer: E. Pulmonary embolism.

This patient has type 1 respiratory failure with severe hypoxia indicating a significant ventilation perfusion mismatch. Pneumonia and atelectasis are unlikely due to the absence of clinical and radiological signs. Similarly, severe sepsis is less likely because of the normal pH and lactate. Acute coronary syndrome complicated with left ventricular failure and pulmonary oedema can result in hypoxia. Pulmonary embolism is the most likely diagnosis given the background of major abdominopelvic cancer surgery with the associated immobilisation, chest pain and unexplained severe hypoxia.

Further reading
1. Tapson VF. Acute pulmonary embolism. *N Engl J Med* 2008; 358: 1037-52.

5   Answer: B. Avoiding nitrous oxide.

During the repair of retinal detachment, the surgeon usually uses intra-ocular injection of air and sulfurhexafluoride (SF6). The coincident use of nitrous oxide expands the volume of air within the eye and increases the intra-ocular pressure. During the procedure nitrous oxide should be discontinued at least 10-15 minutes prior to intra-ocular injection of SF6. Nitrous oxide should be avoided at least 30 days following repair of retinal detachment to prevent a rise in intra-ocular pressure. Rapid sequence induction using succinylcholine can cause a transient increase in intra-ocular pressure but rocuronium can be used as an alternative to succinylcholine.

Further reading
1. Herlich A. Retinal detachment. In: *Clinical cases in anaesthesia*, 3rd ed. Reed AP, Yudkowitz FS, Eds. Philadelphia, USA: Elsevier Churchill Livingstone, 2005; Case 44: 239-41.

6   Answer: B. Anterior to the aorta.

The coeliac plexus consists of the coeliac ganglia with a network of interconnecting nerve fibres supplying the upper abdominal organs (pancreas, liver, gall bladder, stomach, spleen, kidneys, small bowel, and 2/3 of the large bowel). Coeliac ganglia lie on each side of the L1 vertebral body with the aorta lying posteriorly, the pancreas anteriorly and the inferior vena cava laterally. The plexus receives sympathetic fibres from the greater splanchnic nerve (T6 to T10), lesser splanchnic nerve (T10, T11), and least splanchnic nerve (T11, T12).

The block is performed with the patient in the prone position under X-ray guidance. Normally, two needles are inserted, one on each side to block both of the coeliac ganglia; good spread to both sides can sometimes be achieved just using one needle. The needle entry point is just below the tip of the 12th rib. Using X-ray screening in two planes, the needle is advanced until the tip of the needle is in front of the aorta (one needle technique) or just lateral to the aorta (two needle technique) at the level of the L1 vertebra.

Coeliac plexus block relieves pain from non-pelvic intra-abdominal organs. The common indications are to relieve pain related to chronic pancreatitis or carcinoma of the pancreas.

Further reading
1. Garcia-Eroles X, Mayoral V, Montero A, et al. Celiac plexus block: a new technique using the left lateral approach. The Clinical Journal of Pain 2007; 23: 635-7.

7   Answer: A. Transoesophageal Doppler.

A sudden decrease or complete loss of $EtCO_2$ can be due to oesophageal intubation, complete disconnection of the airway, total airway obstruction, cardiac arrest, severe bronchospasm and massive pulmonary embolism or venous air embolism. Venous air embolism (VAE) is a recognised complication of posterior fossa craniotomy in the sitting position. Transoesophageal Doppler and precordial Doppler are sensitive detectors of air in the right atrium, transoesophageal Doppler slightly more so than the precordial Doppler. A mill-wheel murmur can be detected using a precordial stethoscope, but it is a very late sign of VAE. The changes in pulmonary artery wedge pressure also occur at a later stage of VAE. Pulse oximetry may show low oxygen saturation which is not specific for VAE.

Further reading

1. Omlor J. Loss of CO_2 trace. In: *Near misses in neuroanaesthesia.* Russell GB, Cronin AJ, Longo S, Blackburn TW, Eds. Butterworth Heinemann, 2002; Case 6: 19-21.
2. Palmon SC, Moore IE, *et al.* Venous air embolism: a review. *Journal of Clinical Anaesthesia* 1997; 9: 251-7.

8 Answer: B. Negative pressure pulmonary oedema.

This patient remained in respiratory distress despite successful management of the laryngospasm. The most likely diagnosis is either aspiration of gastric contents or negative pressure pulmonary oedema (NPPE). Since the condition improved rapidly after application of CPAP and diuretics it is unlikely to be due to aspiration. There is no history of asthma (ASA1 patient) and there is no mention of bronchodilators in the treatment.

NPPE occurs rarely in patients, requiring active intervention for acute upper airway obstruction during anaesthesia. The risk factors include obesity with obstructive sleep apnoea, the presence of airway lesions, upper airway surgery and young male athletes.

High negative intrathoracic pressures initiate a cascade of events in the development of NPPE. Forceful inspiration against a closed glottis, such as in laryngospasm, can result in markedly negative intrathoracic pressures, up to -140cm H_2O from a baseline average of -4cm H_2O. With such negative intrathoracic pressure, venous return is increased to the right heart, subsequently raising pulmonary hydrostatic pressure. The increased pulmonary hydrostatic pressure leads to the transudation of fluid from the pulmonary capillaries into the pulmonary interstitial space, resulting in pulmonary oedema. Hypoxic vasoconstriction of both pulmonary and systemic arterioles raises systemic blood pressure and increases the afterload of the left and right ventricles.

Expiration against a closed system generates high intraluminal airway pressures. This serves as auto-PEEP (positive end-expiratory pressure) that prevents fluid from leaving the pulmonary capillaries and from entering the alveoli. When laryngospasm is relieved, either spontaneously or by reintubation, the resultant drop in airway pressure causes a transudation of fluid into the alveoli and severe acute pulmonary oedema.

Treatment of NPPE is supportive and includes maintenance of a patent airway and adequate oxygenation. In severe cases, endotracheal intubation and mechanical ventilation with PEEP may be necessary.

Further reading

1. Thiagarajan RR, Laussen PC. Negative pressure pulmonary oedema in children - pathogenesis and clinical management. *Pediatric Anesthesia* 2007; 17: 307-10.
2. Herrick IA, Mahendran B, Penny FJ. Postoperative pulmonary oedema following anesthesia. *J Clin Anesth* 1990; 2: 116-20.
3. Dicpinigaitis PV, Mehta DC. Postobstructive pulmonary oedema induced by endotracheal tube occlusion. *Intensive Care Med* 1995; 21: 1048-50.

9 Answer: D. Amitryptiline.

Amitryptiline is a tricyclic antidepressant. Overdose can present with tachycardia, mydriasis, hyper-reflexia, seizures, coma, ECG changes, hypotension and arrhythmias.

It acts by sodium channel blockade (class 1a anti-arrhythmic drug). ECG changes are a useful measure of toxicity with a QRS duration >120ms indicating a risk of seizures and arrhythmias. A QRS duration >160ms suggests a particularly high risk, but a normal ECG does not exclude significant toxicity. There is no specific antidote. Treatment options include activated charcoal to reduce absorption, sodium bicarbonate to alkalinise blood, which increases protein-binding therefore reducing the free drug concentration, and benzodiazepines for seizures. Phenytoin is the anti-arrhythmic of choice where bicarbonate fails. Supportive measures including sedation and ventilation may be required until the drug is metabolised, usually within 24 hours.

Fluoxetine is a selective serotonin reuptake inhibitor. The most common clinical features after an overdose include agitation, tremor, mild hypertension, arrhythmias and nystagmus. In combination with other drugs such as cocaine, tricyclics and MAOIs, it may produce serotonin syndrome, characterised by a triad of neuromuscular irritability, altered mental status and autonomic instability.

Ethyl glycol poisoning results in metabolic acidosis with an increased anion gap. Amphetamine overdose results in hyperthermia due to its effect on the thermoregulatory centre. It also causes tachycardia, hypertension and arrhythmias due to its sympathomimetic effect.

Further reading
1. Drug overdose. In: *Key topics in critical care*, 2nd ed. Craft TM, Nolan JP, Parr MJA, Eds. Taylor and Francis, 2004.
2. Ward C, Sair M. Oral poisoning: an update. *British Journal of Anaesthesia CEACCP* 2010; 10: 6-10.

10 Answer: D. Anterior spinal artery syndrome.

Anterior spinal artery syndrome (ASAS) occurs due to inadequate blood supply to the anterior 2/3 of the spinal cord. It is characterized by a lower motor neurone type of lesion with reduced or absent pain and temperature sensation below the level of the lesion. The vibration and proprioception (joint position sensation) are, however, preserved because, they are carried by the posterior columns of the spinal cord (supplied by the posterior spinal artery). The blood supply to the anterior 2/3 of the spinal cord is reinforced by the anterior radicular arteries. The largest radicular artery, the artery of Adamkiewicz, usually arises from the aorta at the level of T8-T11 (may vary from T8-L4). There is an increased risk of damage to this radicular artery during major thoraco-abdominal surgical procedures, such as aneurysm repair and oesophagectomy. Other causes include aortic disease (atherosclerosis of the aorta and dissecting aortic aneurysm), hyper-coagulability, acute transverse myelitis, arteriovenous malformation, sickle cell disease and acute transverse myelitis.

Further radiological investigation is essential to rule out other causes of paraplegia such as epidural abscess and haematoma, which are less likely on the third postoperative day. Further clinical signs such as pyrexia and a raised white cell count would support the diagnosis of an epidural abscess.

The posterior spinal artery suplies the posterior 1/3 of the spinal cord, mainly the dorsal columns. Ischaemia of the posterior 1/3 of the spinal cord is less common than the anterior 2/3.

Further reading

1. Djurberg H. Haddad M. Anterior spinal artery syndrome. Paraplegia following segmental ischaemic injury to the spinal cord after oesophagectomy. *Anaesthesia* 1995; 50: 345-8.
2. Sinha AC, Cheung AT. Spinal cord protection and thoracic aortic surgery. *Current Opinion in Anaesthesiology* 2010; 23: 95-102.

11 Answer: D. Deep peroneal and superficial peroneal, and posterior tibial nerves.

Ankle block is a safe and effective method for providing analgesia following surgical procedures on bones and soft tissues of the foot and can also be used alone as a regional technique. Five nerve branches carry sensation from the different areas of the foot. All are branches of the sciatic nerve, except the saphenous nerve, which is the terminal branch of the femoral nerve. The sciatic nerve divides into the tibial nerve and the common peroneal nerve at a variable point between the buttock and the popliteal fossa. The tibial nerve then divides into the posterior tibial and sural nerves, and the common peroneal nerve into the deep and superficial peroneal nerves. The posterior tibial nerve finally divides into the medial and lateral plantar nerves. The medial plantar nerve provides sensory innervation to the plantar aspect of the great toe, the deep peroneal nerve innervates the first web space and the superficial peroneal nerve innervates the medial half of the dorsal aspect of the great toe. All three nerves therefore need to be blocked for great toe amputation.

Further reading

1. Reilley TE, Gerhardt MA. Anesthesia for foot and ankle surgery. *Clin Podiatr Med Surg* 2002; 19: 125-47.

12 Answer: A. I.M. carboprost 250µg repeated at 15-minute intervals if necessary.

Carboprost has been successfully used following failure of conventional treatment. It is not licensed for intra-myometrial use. The uterus after delivery is extremely vascular and an intra-myometrial injection may cause systemic adverse affects. The BNF recommended dose of oxytocin after a Caesarean section is 5 units I.V. followed by an infusion if necessary. Rectal administration of drugs can be unreliable in a shocked patient. In the non-shocked patient, misoprostol is often used at a dose of 800µg per rectally at the end of the operation to maintain uterine tone.

Further reading
1. Howell C, Irani S. Massive obstetric haemorrhage. In: *MOET course manual*, 2nd ed. Royal College of Obstetrics & Gynaecology (RCOA) Press, 2007; Chapter 17: 179.

13 Answer: E. Maintenance of a normal to high heart rate avoiding sudden bradycardia, and maintenance of a normal to low SVR.

General anaesthesia is usually the technique of choice in patients with mitral regurgitation. Although a decrease in systemic vascular resistance (SVR) is beneficial, an uncontrolled or sudden response can be detrimental. The main aim is to avoid events that may further decrease cardiac output. Maintenance of a normal to slightly increased heart rate is recommended, as forward left ventricular stroke volume is likely to be heart rate-dependent. Likewise, any sudden increase in systemic vascular resistance will increase the regurgitant fraction and thereby reduce the forward flow.

Further reading
1. Valvular heart disease. In: *Anesthesia and co-existing diseases*, 4th ed. Stoelting RK, Dierdorf S, Eds. Philadelphia, USA: Churchill Livingstone, 2002; Chapter 2: 33-5.

14   Answer: E. Pericarditis.

The presenting features of pericariditis include retrosternal stabbing chest pain, a low-grade intermittent fever, shortness of breath, a cough and dyspnoea. The most common clinical finding is a pericardial rub. Serous pericarditis is commonly seen in rheumatoid arthritis and systemic lupus erythematosus (SLE). The other causes of acute pericarditis include viral infection, tuberculosis and scleroderma. Acute pericarditis with a pericardial effusion may occur following myocardial infarction and trauma such as cardiac surgery and pacemaker insertion.

The classical signs of cardiac tamponade include an elevated JVP, hypotension and muffled heart sounds. Signs of right and left ventricular failure can be seen in patients with cardiac tamponade. The clinical features of congestive cardiac failure include peripheral oedema, ascites and raised JVP. In pericarditis, superficial inflammation of the myocardium results in diffuse ST segment elevation on the ECG. Absence of reciprocal ST segment depression on the ECG distinguishes acute pericarditis from acute myocardial infarction.

Further reading
1. Pericardial Diseases. In: *Anesthesia and co-existing disease*, 4th ed. Stoelting RK, Dierdorf SF, Eds. Philadelphia, USA: Churchill Livingstone, 2002; 135-42.

15   Answer: B. Her operative mortality is about 25%.

In patients with liver disease the mortality risk can be estimated using Pugh's modification of Child's scoring system. There are five variables in the scoring system (Table 1). Each variable has a lowest score of 1 and a highest score of 3. From the available clinical and laboratory data, this patient has a total score of 8. This patient therefore carries a moderate peri-operative risk with a mortality rate of about 25%.

Variable	Score		
	1	2	3
Encephalopathy	None ✓	Minimal	Advanced
Ascites	None ✓	Minimal	Moderate
Bilirubin, mg/dL	<2	2-3 ✓	>3
Albumin, g/L	>35	28-35 ✓	<28
PT (s above control)	<4	4-6 ✓	>6

Table 1. Pugh's modification of Child's score.

(Encephalopathy: minimal = grade 1 and 2; advanced = grade 3 and 4)

Total score versus risk

Total score	Child's class	Operative mortality
5-6	A	Low, <5%
7-9	B	Moderate, 25%
10-15	C	High, >50%

Further reading
1. Diseases of the liver and biliary tract. In: *Anesthesia and co-existing diseases*, 4th ed, Stoelting RK, Dierdorf S, Eds. Philadelphia, USA: Churchill Livingstone, 2002; Chapter 18: 299-324.
2. Vaja R, McNicol R, Sisley I. Anaesthesia for patients with liver disease. *British Journal of Anaesthesia* 2010; 10: 15-9.

16 Answer: D. Posterior angle of the rib.

The intercostal nerve enters the subcostal groove and continues to run parallel to the rib. Its course within the thorax is sandwiched between internal intercostal and innermost intercostal muscles. A typical intercostal nerve gives off the lateral cutaneous branch and terminates as the anterior cutaneous nerve.

The lateral cutaneous branch of an intercostal nerve is given off at variable points distal to the posterior axillary line. So, for reliable blockade of the lateral cutaneous branch, the intercostal nerve should be blocked at the posterior angle of the rib. 3ml of local anesthetic solution injected through a needle spreads some 4-6cm easily along that single subcostal groove distally and proximally. If a catheter is inserted at the angle of the rib and directed medially 2-3cm, a larger volume (about 20ml) of solution could be injected which can spread to the paravertebral space to block 3-5 intercostal nerves.

Further reading
1. Karmakar MK, Ho AMH. Acute pain management of patients with multiple fractured ribs. *J Trauma* 2003; 54: 612-5.

17 Answer: D. Idiopathic pulmonary hypertension.

Idiopathic pulmonary hypertension (IPH) is defined as a mean pulmonary artery pressure greater than 25mm Hg at rest with a normal pulmonary capillary wedge pressure and the absence of identifiable causes of pulmonary hypertension. The exact pathogenesis of IPH is unclear. The mechanism that appears to be most widely accepted is that of pulmonary vasoconstriction with an imbalance of vasoactive mediators. Factors such as thromboxane, arachidonic acid metabolites, and prostacyclin, as well as other endothelial factors, have been invoked. Trigger factors such as high altitude, hypoxaemia, drugs, toxins, sympathetic tone, and autoimmune disorders, can cause pulmonary vasoconstriction in susceptible individuals.

Morbidity and mortality rates vary and depend on the age, the degree of pulmonary hypertension, and the response to vasodilator therapy. Death as a result of both acute and chronic right heart failure and its associated arrhythmias may occur. The treatment of IPH includes general medical measures such as annual influenza vaccination, treating fever and respiratory illnesses aggressively, and supplemental oxygen. Patients with severe pulmonary hypertension resulting in recurrent syncope or right-to-left intracardiac shunting may benefit from palliation with blade atrial septostomy or balloon dilation of the atrial septum.

The rationale for the use of vasodilators in patients with IPH is to counteract vasoconstriction. The various drugs used are oral calcium channel blockers (e.g. nifedipine) and continuous intravenous prostacyclin. The latter may be recommended for the patient with right heart failure and/or symptoms that may include syncope. Endothelin receptor blockers and phosphodiesterase-5 inhibitors have also been advocated.

Further reading
1. Rashid A, Ivy D. Severe paediatric pulmonary hypertension: new management strategies. *Arch Dis Child* 2005; 90(1): 92-8.
2. Melson H, Sykes E, *et al*. Perioperative implications of pulmonary hypertension. *CPD Anaesthesia* 2008; 10: 39-66.

119

18   Answer: C. Hydralazine and magnesium.

This lady has severe pre-eclampsia with a diastolic blood pressure ≥110mmHg and systolic blood pressure ≥170mmHg with significant proteinuria (3+ is approximately equal to 3g/L). The presence of any of the following clinical features constitutes severe pre-eclampsia (in addition to hypertension and proteinuria):

◆   Symptoms of severe headache.
◆   Visual disturbance.
◆   Liver tenderness.
◆   Platelet count falling to below 100×10^6/L.
◆   Epigastric pain and/or vomiting.
◆   Abnormal liver enzymes (ALT or AST rising to above 70I.U./L).
◆   Clonus.
◆   HELLP syndrome.
◆   Papilloedema.

Antihypertensive treatment should be started in women with a systolic blood pressure over 160mmHg or a diastolic blood pressure over 110mmHg or other markers of severe disease. Labetalol should be avoided in women with known asthma.

Hydralazine can be used for the acute management of severe hypertension.

In addition to hydralazine, magnesium is likely to be beneficial in view of the signs of cerebral irritability and prevention of eclampsia. The patient should be closely monitored, treated with antihypertensives and stabilised, and delivery should be considered depending on the maternal response to treatment and foetal age.

Further reading
1. RCOG Green-Top 10A guideline: The management of severe pre-eclampsia/eclampsia. (www.rcog.org.uk).

19   Answer: B. Tension pneumothorax.

The two main complications of positive pressure ventilation in a patient with asthma are pneumothorax and haemodynamic collapse. The reported incidence of pneumothorax during manual ventilation following endotracheal intubation is as high as 75%. During manual bagging extremely high airway pressures can be generated. To prevent a pneumothorax, slow rate low tidal volume ventilation should be used. Sepsis and myocardial infarction are also possible diagnoses. Patients with severe asthma usually present with tachycardia and hypertension due to increased sympathetic drive and release of catecholamine. Associated fever, hyperventilation and sweating can lead to dehydration and hypovolaemia. Consequently, soon after sedation is administered, the vasodilatory effect of sedation and reduced catecholamine levels can result in cardiovascular collapse.

Further reading
1. De Mendoza D, Lujan M, Rello J. Mechanical ventilation for asthma Exacerbations. In: *Yearbook of intensive care medicine*. Vincent LL, Eds. New York, USA: Springer, 2008; VII: 256-68.
2. Rodrigo GJ, Rodrigo C, Hall JB. Acute asthma in adults: a review. *Chest* 2004; 125: 1081-102.

20   Answer: A. Intravenous dexamethasone.

Insertion of a nasogastric tube can result in oropharyngeal trauma. In this patient it resulted in trauma to the uvula and subsequent oedema leading to difficulty in breathing. The other cause of trauma to the uvula could have been from the blind Yankauer suction. Dexamethasone is the treatment of choice for uvular oedema. The anti-inflammatory potency of dexamethasone is 30 times greater than hydrocortisone. Dexamethasone also has a long half-life of 36-72 hours. Steroids decrease the capillary permeability and therefore reduce the oedema. I.V. hydrocortisone is less effective than dexamethasone in reducing oedema.

Further reading
1. Holden JP, Vaughn WC, Brock-Utne JG. Airway complications following functional endoscopic sinus surgery. *J Clinical Anesthesia* 2002; 14: 154-7.
2. Postoperative airway complications after sinus surgery. In: *Clinical anesthesia: near misses and lessons learned*. Brock-Utne JG, Ed. New York, USA: Springer, 2008; Case 22: 54-6.
3. Hawkins DB, Crockett DM, Shum TK. Corticosteroids in airway management. *Otolaryn Head Neck Surg* 1983; 91: 593-6.

21 Answer: C. Amputation of limb.

Chronic post-surgical pain (CPSP) is a serious and relatively common complication following surgery. It is defined as pain occurring after a surgical procedure, at least 2 months after the procedure, when no other cause for the pain can be found (e.g. malignancy, infection). The incidence of CPSP following specific surgical procedures is shown in Table 2.

Table 2. The incidence of chronic post-surgical pain (CPSP) following specific surgical procedures.

Cholecystectomy	3-56%
Mastectomy	11-57%
Amputation of limb	30-85%
Thoracotomy	5-67%
Hernia repair	0-63%

Further reading
1. Searle RD, Simpson KH. Chronic post-surgical pain. *British Journal of Anaesthesia CEACCP* 2010; 10: 12-4.

22   Answer: B. Haloperidol 0.5-1mg I.V.

The most likely diagnosis is postoperative delirium (POD). The incidence in elderly patients with hip fracture is high, ranging from 16-62% with an average of 35%. The primary treatment is identification and correction of any underlying causes such as pain, hypoxia and dehydration. Pharmacological treatment may be necessary when agitation puts the patient and staff at risk of harm.

Haloperidol is the drug of choice for treating POD. It is administered at a dose of 0.5-1mg I.V. every 5-10 minutes until the agitation is controlled. It has a long half-life of up to 72 hours; it is therefore essential to titrate the dose carefully to avoid over sedation. Benzodiazepines such as midazolam and diazepam can result in sedation, respiratory depression and hypoxia, which may aggravate agitation. In patients undergoing cardiac surgery, ketamine has been shown to reduce the incidence of POD when administered at a dose of 0.5mg/kg at induction.

Further reading.
1. Deiner S, Silverstein JH. Postoperative delirium and cognitive dysfunction. *British Journal of Anaesthesia* 2009; 103 (Suppl. I): i41-6.

23   Answer: D. Uterine atony.

The most common cause for intra and postpartum haemorrhage following prolonged labour is uterine atony. Other less common causes include a retained placenta, other causes of mechanical obstruction to contraction, and genital tract trauma. Rarer causes include coagulopathies, endometritis and intra-uterine sepsis.

Further reading
1. RCOG Green-Top 10A guideline: The management of severe pre-eclampsia/eclampsia. (www.rcog.org.uk).

24 Answer: A. Platelet count of 102 x 10⁹/L 6 days after starting heparin.

It is important to distinguish heparin-induced thrombocytopaenia (HIT) from other causes of a low platelet count. HIT usually occurs 5 days after starting heparin, unless the patient has been exposed to heparin in the previous 30 days, in which case it can occur immediately. HIT is characterized by a fall in the platelet count to less than 50% of its previous level. Extremely low platelet counts (typically $<15 \times 10^9$/L) are not usually associated with HIT.

Not all platelet-heparin antibodies are associated with the development of HIT. Only 1% of patients with detectable antibodies will develop clinically relevant disease. IgA and IgM antibodies are unimportant - only those with IgG antibodies will develop the disease.

In true HIT the platelet count will start to recover 2 to 3 days after stopping heparin, and is usually normal by day 14. A recovery more rapid than this does not support the diagnosis of HIT.

Other causes of thrombocytopaenia must be ruled out in order for the diagnosis of HIT to be made. Disseminated intravascular coagulation (DIC) is associated with severe sepsis and will lead to consumption of platelets. A low fibrinogen level supports the diagnosis of DIC rather than HIT.

Further reading
1. Hall A, Thachil J, Martlew V. Heparin-induced thrombocytopenia in the intensive care unit. *J Intensive Care Soc* 2010; 11: 20-5.

25 Answer: E. Mallory-Weiss syndrome.

Mallory-Weiss syndrome is upper gastro-intestinal bleeding due to linear mucosal tears at the gastro-oesophageal junction, and typically occurs following episodes of retching and vomiting. There is usually a history of excessive alcohol intake preceding the episode of vomiting. Massive bleeding is uncommon in reflux oesophagitis and acute gastritis. The history of alcohol abuse and absence of occult blood in the stool differentiates Mallory-Weiss syndrome from a bleeding peptic ulcer. A history of epigastric pain and the passage of black stools (melaena) suggest peptic ulcer disease. A hiatus hernia can cause reflux oesophagitis. Reflux oesophagitis usually causes epigastric pain which often radiates to the back.

Further reading

1. Diseases of the gastro-intestinal system. In: *Anesthesia and co-existing diseases*, 4th ed. Stoelting RK, Dierdorf S, Eds. Philadelphia, USA: Churchill Livingstone, 2002; Chapter 19: 337-8.

26 Answer: B. Stellate ganglion block.

This patient has refractory angina. The various treatment options for this condition include analgesic drugs such as opioids, TENS therapy, stellate ganglion block, and spinal cord stimulation. In this patient opioids may not be safe as he suffers from obstructive sleep apnoea. TENS therapy is contraindicated due to the presence of a pacemaker. Refractory angina pain is vascular pain and responds poorly to NSAIDs. A stellate ganglion block is therefore the most suitable option in this patient.

The stellate ganglion is formed by the fusion of the inferior cervical and the first thoracic ganglion as they meet at the neck of the first rib. It is present in 80% of subjects. The structures anterior to the ganglion include the skin and subcutaneous tissue, the sternocleidomastoid and the carotid sheath. The dome of the lung lies anterior and inferior to the ganglion. The prevertebral fascia, vertebral body of C7, oesophagus and thoracic duct lie medially. Structures posterior to the ganglion include the longus colli muscle, anterior scalene muscle, vertebral artery, brachial plexus sheath and neck of the first rib.

The indications for a stellate ganglion block include complex regional pain syndrome types I and II, refractory angina, phantom limb pain, post-herpetic neuralgia and vascular insufficiency, such as Raynaud's syndrome.

A successful stellate ganglion block is indicated by the development of Horner's syndrome. The classic clinical findings associated with Horner's syndrome are ptosis, enophthalmos, pupillary miosis and facial anhidrosis. The benefits of stellate ganglion block may only be temporary; the duration of analgesia is very variable.

Further reading

1. Chester M, Hammond C, Leach A. Long-term benefits of stellate ganglion block in severe chronic refractory angina. *Pain* 2000; 87: 103-5.

27 Answer: A. The axillary nerve.

The axillary nerve arises from the posterior cord of the brachial plexus and carries nerve fibres from C5 and C6. It travels through a quadrilateral space bounded above by teres major, below by teres minor, medially by the long head of triceps and laterally by the surgical neck of the humerus. It divides into anterior and posterior branches. The anterior branch of the axillary nerve winds round the surgical neck of the humerus. The axillary nerve provides sensory innervation to the lower part of the deltoid region and motor innervation to the deltoid and teres minor muscles. Weakness of the deltoid limits abduction of the arm (0-30°). Contraction of supraspinatus causes initial abduction up to 30°, and further abduction from 30-90° is achieved by contraction of the deltoid.

The median nerve supplies the pronator teres and flexors of the wrist except flexor carpi ulnaris and part of flexor digitorum profundus. Median nerve injury above the level of the elbow results in weakness of pronation and flexion of the wrist.

The suprascapular nerve supplies the supraspinatus and infraspinatus muscles. Injury to the musculocutaneous nerve results in weakness of flexion of the forearm (biceps brachii, coracobrachialis and brachialis). Radial nerve injury results in weakness of extension at the elbow and wrist.

Further reading

1. Kroll DA, Caplan RA, Posner K, *et al*. Nerve injury associated with anesthesia. *Anesthesiology* 1990; 73: 202-7.

28 Answer: D. Ruptured abdominal aortic aneurysm.

The majority of abdominal aortic aneurysms (AAA) are asymptomatic and are incidentally discovered during routine physical examination or during an unrelated diagnostic imaging study.

The classic triad of ruptured AAA is hypotension, a pulsatile abdominal mass, and flank or back pain. Back pain is the most common symptom, due to leak of blood into the retroperitoneal space. The combination of a past history of aneurysm and the sudden onset of severe back ache should lead to the diagnosis of ruptured aortic aneurysm.

Pain in the right hypochondrium and at the inferior angle of the right scapula is common in cholecystitis. In pancreatitis, pain is in the epigastric region, and often radiates to the back. In severe acute pancreatitis the patient may present in shock. Nausea and vomiting are common; there may be a past history of dyspepsia, biliary colic or transient jaundice. In lumbar disc prolapse, the back pain usually radiates to the legs and shock is uncommon.

Further reading
1. Tan WA, Makaroun MS. Abdominal aortic aneurysm rupture. (http://emedicine.medscape.com/article/416397-overview).

29 Answer: C. Serum calcium.

A rapid decrease in serum calcium can produce skeletal muscle spasm manifesting as laryngospasm. The parathyroid glands may be accidentally removed or may be injured during total thyroidectomy resulting in hypocalcaemia. The serum thyroid stimulating hormone (TSH) level is not usually altered immediately following this surgery. TSH measurement may be needed at a later stage to assess thyroid replacement therapy. Hypocalcaemia can result in a prolonged QT interval on the ECG but this is not a reliable guide to the presence of hypocalcaemia.

Hypoalbuminaemia results in low measured serum calcium but the ionised calcium can be normal. Other causes include acute pancreatitis, vitamin D deficiency, hypomagnesaemia, malnutrition, sepsis, parathyroidectomy and renal failure. Hyperventilation and metabolic alkalosis result in low ionised calcium.

The clinical signs and symptoms of hypocalcaemia are caused by increased neuronal irritability leading to neurological, respiratory, cardiovascular and psychiatric manifestations. Neurological manifestations include paraesthesia of the distal extremities and circum-oral area, Chvostek's and Trousseau's signs, muscle cramps, tetany, and seizures. Acute hypocalcaemia can result in laryngospasm and bronchospasm, particularly after parathyroidectomy. Cardiovascular manifestations include hypotension, bradycardia and precipitation of digitalis toxicity.

Further reading

1. Aguilera IM, Vaughan RS. Calcium and anaesthetist. *Anaesthesia* 2001; 55: 779-90.
2. Water, electrolyte and acid-base disturbances. In: *Anesthesia and co-existing diseases*, 4th ed. Stoelting RK, Dierdorf S, Eds. Philadelphia, USA: Churchill Livingstone, 2002; Chapter 21: 385-90.

30 Answer: B. Lingual nerve.

The lingual nerve is a branch of the mandibular nerve, and carries the fibres from the chorda tympani (branch of the facial nerve). The lingual nerve provides sensory innervation to the mucous membrane of the anterior two-thirds of the tongue, and to the side wall and floor of the mouth. The fibres from the chorda tympani are secretomotor to the submandibular and sublingual salivary glands and also carry taste sensation from the anterior two-thirds of the tongue.

The inferior alveolar nerve is the largest branch of the mandibular nerve. It provides sensory innervation to the molar teeth and premolar teeth.

The glossopharyngeal nerve carries sensation from the pharynx, the tonsillar region and the posterior one third of the tongue. It provides motor innervation to the stylopharyngeus muscle and to the secretomotor fibres of the parotid gland. It also innervates the carotid sinus and body.

The buccal nerve supplies the skin over the anterior part of the cheek, the mucous membrane of the inner aspect of the cheek and the lateral aspect of the gum adjacent to the molar teeth of the mandible.

The hypoglossal nerve supplies all the intrinsic and extrinsic muscles of the tongue (with the exception of palatoglossus).

Further reading

1. The cranial nerves. In: *Anatomy for anaesthetists*. 8th ed. Ellis H, Feldman S, Harrop-Griffiths W. Oxford: Blackwell Science Ltd, 2004; Part 6: 235-83.
2. Graff-Radford SB, Evans RW. Lingual nerve injury. (http://www.medscape.com/viewarticle/462066).

Set 5 questions

1   A 44-year-old female presents with generalized body pain. She feels lethargic and also complains of depression. She has generalized muscle tenderness all over her body. She is known to have irritable bowel syndrome. What is the most likely diagnosis?

a.   Muscular dystrophy.
b.   Polymyalgia rheumatica.
c.   Fibromyalgia.
d.   Chronic fatigue syndrome.
e.   Rheumatoid arthritis.

2   A 26-year-old primigravida diagnosed with severe pre-eclampsia was treated with magnesium sulphate. She subsequently had a Caesarean section performed under epidural anaesthesia. No adverse events were recorded intra-operatively and she was transferred to the high dependency unit where she was making a good recovery. 24 hours later she becomes lethargic and confused. She has reduced muscle tone and reflexes. Her ECG shows a prolonged P-R interval and widened QRS. What is the most likely diagnosis?

a.   Pulmonary embolism.
b.   Amniotic fluid embolism.
c.   Hypermagnesaemia.
d.   Hyponatraemia.
e.   Hyperkalaemia.

3   A 78-year-old man underwent a hemi-arthroplasty of the left hip under general anaesthesia. He was given atropine in recovery for severe bradycardia. Following this he become extremely restless, agitated and confused. Which of the following is likely to be the most suitable treatment for this patient's restlessness and agitation?

a.   Intravenous midazolam.
b.   Intravenous physostigmine.
c.   Intravenous neostigmine.
d.   Intravenous haloperidol.
e.   Oral clonidine.

4   A 46-year-old male patient is admitted to the high dependency unit following severe myalgia, diarrhoea, sweating, cough and fever with a temperature of 39.1°C. He is fit and well otherwise and has a history of recent travel abroad on a business trip. A diagnosis of severe community-acquired pneumonia is made and culture yields a gram negative bacillus. Which of these organisms is most likely to be the cause of his infection?

a.   *Streptococcus pneumoniae.*
b.   *Legionella pneumophilia.*
c.   *Staphylococcus aureus.*
d.   *Haemophilus influenzae.*
e.   *Mycoplasma pneumoniae.*

5   A 66-year-old female is scheduled for major surgery. She suffers from Parkinson's disease for which she is treated with levodopa. She has a history of PONV. Which of the following anti-emetic regimes would be most suitable for this patient?

a.   Domperidone and ondansetron.
b.   Metoclopramide and ondansetron.
c.   Droperidol and prochlorperazine.
d.   Ondansetron and prochlorperazine.
e.   Prochlorperazine and metoclopramide.

6 A 72-year-old male who is a chronic smoker complains of constant leg pain. Clinical examination has revealed ischaemic ulcers in both his legs. He has been assessed by a vascular surgeon and has been referred to the pain clinic for the management of his pain. Which of the below is likely to be the most effective treatment for his pain?

a. Lumbar epidural steroids.
b. Nerve root block.
c. Chemical lumbar sympathectomy.
d. Regular morphine.
e. Superior hypogastric plexus block.

7 A 30-year-old male patient is undergoing a laparoscopic cholecystectomy. Halfway through the surgery, despite adequate inspired oxygen and ventilation, his SpO_2 decreases to 90%. Clinical examination reveals distended neck veins, and reduced movement and breath sounds on the left side of the chest. What should be the next step in the management of this patient?

a. Increasing minute ventilation.
b. Arterial blood gas analysis.
c. Endotracheal suction.
d. Needle decompression and insertion of a chest drain.
e. Application of PEEP.

8 A 65-year-old male patient with a history of heavy smoking presents with chest pain and a cough of 2 months' duration. On clinical examination there are enlarged supraclavicular lymph nodes on the left side. Chest X-ray demonstrates a 2cm lesion in the left upper lobe. The biochemistry reveals normal potassium, urea and creatinine but serum sodium is 124mmol/L. Which of following is the most likely cause for his hyponatraemia?

a. Cerebral salt wasting syndrome.
b. Small cell carcinoma of the lung.
c. Adrenal insufficiency.
d. Hypothyroidism.
e. Pulmonary tuberculosis.

9 A 58-year-old gentleman with a history of recent recovery from a flu-like illness has been admitted to the medical ward with a history of progressive ascending weakness of the lower limbs with preserved bladder function. On examination he has flaccid paralysis and peripheral neuropathy in the lower limbs. CSF examination shows a normal cell count but a raised protein concentration. The most likely diagnosis is:

a. Myasthenia gravis.
b. Transverse myelitis.
c. Severe electrolyte disturbances.
d. Motor neurone disease.
e. Guillain-Barré syndrome.

10 A 70-year-old male patient is scheduled for a right carotid endarterectomy under a cervical plexus block. A deep cervical plexus block is performed using 12ml of 0.5% levobupivacaine. Five minutes after completing the injection, the patient complains of difficulty in breathing and soon becomes unconscious and apnoeic requiring intubation and ventilation. When he is still able to speak he denies circumoral numbness or tingling. The blood pressure decreases from 170/84 to 70/44mm Hg and responds to intravenous fluids and ephedrine. The ECG shows sinus rhythm with a heart rate of 64 bpm. About an hour later the patient wakes up and is extubated. The neurological examination is completely normal and he is cardiovascularly stable. The most likely cause for the respiratory arrest in this patient is:

a. Local anaesthetic toxicity.
b. Epidural block.
c. Subarachnoid block.

d.   Intravascular injection.
e.   Right phrenic nerve palsy.

✗11   A 70-year-old female with myopia is scheduled to have a cataract
operation. She is known to have COAD and has been on a home
nebuliser for the last 6 months. She also takes warfarin for atrial
fibrillation; her most recent INR was 2.2. Which one of the following
is the most appropriate anaesthetic technique?

a.   Retrobulbar block.
b.   Peribulbar block.
c.   Sub-Tenon's block.
d.   General anaesthetic with endotracheal intubation.
e.   General anaesthetic with LMA.

↑12   A 60-year-old man with hypertension presents for an inguinal hernia
repair. His past medical history includes a heart transplant 3 years
before for idiopathic cardiomyopathy. During the intra-operative
period which of the following drugs would be most suitable for
treating bradycardia?

a.   Glycopyrrolate.
b.   Atropine.
c.   Ephedrine.
d.   Isoprenaline.
e.   Norephedrine.

13   For patients presenting for thoracic surgery in which of the following
is the use of a double-lumen tube for lung isolation most strongly
indicated?

a.   Thoracic aortic aneurysm.
b.   Giant unilateral lung cyst.
c.   Lobectomy.
d.   Oesophagectomy.
e.   Spinal thoracic surgery.

⊁ 14 A 37-year-old female patient is admitted to the intensive care unit with shortness of breath and hypotension. Despite vigorous resuscitation, she remains hypotensive. Her heart rate is 110bpm and BP is 92/50mmHg. The results of pulmonary artery flotation catheter measurements are shown in Table 1.

Table 1. Results of pulmonary artery flotation catheter measurements.

RV pressure	PA pressure	PA wedge pressure
65/12mmHg	80/30mmHg	36mmHg

Which of the following drug combinations would be the most appropriate in this patient?

a. Noradrenaline and dobutamine.
b. Noradrenaline and propranolol.
c. Furosemide and dobutamine.
d. Nitroglycerine and dobutamine.
e. Noradrenaline and nitroglycerine. /

✝ 15 A 70-year-old male patient with type II diabetes, hypertension and ischaemic heart disease is undergoing a laparotomy for carcinoma of the sigmoid colon. Which of the following monitors would be the most sensitive detector of intra-operative myocardial ischaemia?

a. Electrocardiography.
b. Transosesophageal echocardiography.
c. Pulmonary capillary wedge pressure measurement.
d. ECG monitoring with CM5 configuration.
e. Dipyridamole-thallium scanning.

16 An 82-year-old lady presents with unilateral burning pain in the T7 dermatome on the right side. She complains of severe pain associated with a tingling and itching sensation. She is unable to tolerate light touch in the area. Her medical history includes hypertension, COAD, and end-stage renal failure. She recently had a course of steroids. What would be the most appropriate initial treatment for her pain?

a. Gabapentin.
b. Amitriptyline.
c. Morphine sulphate.
d. Lidocaine 5% plasters.
e. Capsaicin 0.025% cream.

17 A 47-year-old female is receiving intravenous antibiotic therapy for subacute bacterial endocarditis. She gradually becomes more breathless. Clinical examination reveals a pulse rate of 112/minute, a BP of 118/52mmHg, raised jugular venous pressure and diastolic and systolic murmurs at the left sternal edge. The most likely diagnosis in this patient is:

a. Ruptured aneurysm of the ascending aorta.
b. Mitral stenosis.
c. Cardiac failure.
d. Ruptured valve cusp of the mitral valve.
e. Acute myocardial infarction.

18 A 32-year-old woman with a history of asthma presents to the emergency department with shortness of breath and wheeze. On arrival to the emergency department her respiratory rate is 34/minute with an SpO_2 of 90%. She is immediately given oxygen at 15L/minute followed by nebulised salbutamol 5mg and ipratropium bromide 500µg. Fifteen minutes after the nebulisers have been administered, her respiratory rate is still rapid at 32/minute and her SpO_2 is 92%. Clinical examination reveals no

wheezing. An arterial blood gas measurement shows a PaO_2 of 8kPa and a $PaCO_2$ of 6.5kPa. Which of the following should be performed next?

a.   Rapid sequence induction, intubation and commencement of positive pressure ventilation.
b.   Intravenous salbutamol by infusion at 5µg/min.
c.   Intravenous aminophylline 5mg/kg.
d.   Intravenous magnesium sulphate 2g over 20 minutes.
e.   Administration of Heliox (70:30 helium/oxygen mixture) by face mask.

+19 A 45-year-old patient is undergoing a craniotomy and evacuation of an intracranial haematoma. Anaesthesia is induced and maintained with target-controlled infusions of remifentanil and propofol. An arterial blood sample, prior to craniotomy, has shown a PaO_2 of 42kPa and $PaCO_2$ of 4.7kPa. On opening the skull the neurosurgeon comments that the appearance suggests significantly raised intracranial pressure. Which of the following therapeutic options should be carried out first to reduce the ICP?

a.   Intravenous infusion of mannitol 0.5g/kg.
b.   Intravenous administration of 8mg of dexamethasone.
c.   Use of a vasopressor infusion to achieve a mean arterial pressure of 90mmHg.
d.   Administration of 0.9% saline to achieve a haematocrit of 30%.
e.   Increase in minute volume to achieve a $PaCO_2$ of 3.5kPa.

20 A 37-year-old man presents for surgery on his hand. He has no medical problems, and wants to have his surgery done under a regional block. A brachial plexus block via the axillary approach is performed using a total of 30ml of 0.375% levobupivacaine. The block is tested before the start of surgery. Sensation is maintained over the thumb and posterior surface of the hand, but there is good anaesthesia over the rest of the hand. How should this situation be managed?

a. Conversion to general anaesthesia.
b. Repeat the axillary brachial plexus block with the same dose of local anaesthetic.
c. Fentanyl 1μg/kg by intravenous injection.
d. Infiltration of 5ml 0.5% levobupivacaine at the elbow between the brachioradialis and the biceps tendon.
e. Midazolam 2-3mg by intravenous injection.

21 A 42-year-old male has been suffering from radicular pain in the L4 nerve distribution of his right leg. He had a discectomy at the L4/L5 level 2 years ago; his pain, however, still remains a significant problem. He has tried neuropathic and opioid medications, TENS, a lumbar epidural and physiotherapy without satisfactory pain relief. TENS relieves his pain for a short duration only. He works as a security officer and is quite keen to continue working. His family and employer are sympathetic and supportive. What would be the next most suitable therapy for his pain?

a. Cognitive behavioural therapy.
b. Physiotherapy.
c. Intrathecal drug delivery using opioids.
d. Spinal cord stimulation.
e. Acupuncture.

22 A 73-year-old man is undergoing an emergency laparotomy for a perforated duodenal ulcer. His blood pressure is low at 73/46mm Hg, and his heart rate is 103 bpm. Which one of these clinical measurements would suggest that he is likely to respond to a fluid bolus?

a. Central venous pressure of 9mmHg.
b. Pulmonary capillary wedge pressure of 16mmHg.
c. Stroke volume variation of 12%.
d. Urine output of 18ml in the last hour.
e. Capillary refill time of 5 seconds.

23

A 63-year-old woman is receiving a continuous epidural infusion of local anaesthetic for analgesia following gastrectomy. It is the second postoperative day. She is pain-free but complains of loss of sensation in her legs as well as motor block. On examination she has a sensory block from T4-S5 on both sides. There is a dense motor block in both lower limbs. Her temperature is 36.5°C. The clinical record reveals that the patient is receiving 20mg of enoxaparin once daily and her INR is 1.1. What should be your next course of action?

a. Reassure the patient that everything is normal.
b. Stop the epidural infusion and reassess after 2 hours.
c. Give 2 units of fresh frozen plasma.
d. Prescribe intravenous flucloxacillin 2g 6-hourly.
e. Arrange an immediate MRI scan of the spine.

24

A 24-year-old female presents to the emergency department with confusion, tachycardia and convulsions gradually worsening for the past 2 hours. She has a history of drug abuse and has been recently started on citalopram for depression. Which of the following would be the most appropriate immediate management?

a. Lorazepam 4mg I.V.
b. Activated charcoal.
c. Cyproheptadine.
d. 225mmol of 8.4% sodium bicarbonate.
e. Haemodialysis.

25

A 3-year-old boy is brought to the accident and emergency department by his parents with a 1-week history of malaise and excessive thirst. He is drowsy but responsive to voice. His respiratory rate is 50 breaths per minute, heart rate is 180 bpm and BP is 70/40mm Hg. Initial investigations reveal serum glucose 25mmol/L, sodium 130mmol/L, potassium 4.0mmol/L, pH 7.08 and lactate 3.1mmol/L. The appropriate initial treatment is:

a. Intravenous insulin bolus.
b. Intravenous bicarbonate.
c. 20ml/kg Hartmann's solution.
d. 10ml/kg of 0.9% saline.
e. Mannitol 0.5g/kg.

26 A 28-year pregnant woman in her first trimester undergoes surgery for a left tibial fracture following a road traffic accident. On the third postoperative day she develops swelling and pain in the right calf. A deep vein thrombosis (DVT) is suspected and confirmed following a Doppler scan. What is the most appropriate treatment for this condition in this patient?

a. 5000 units of unfractionated heparin subcutaneously twice a day.
b. Intravenous heparin infusion.
c. Oral warfarin therapy.
d. Placement of an inferior vena caval filter.
e. Enoxaparin 1mg/kg subcutaneously every 12 hours.

27 A 52-year-old woman is brought into the emergency department with a history of shortness of breath and central chest pain. She was discharged home 5 days before following a total knee replacement. On clinical examination she is hypoxic and tachycardic and her BP is 86/45mm Hg following infusion of 1L of Hartmann's solution. Which of the following would be the most suitable diagnostic test for pulmonary embolism?

a. Troponin.
b. Echocardiography.
c. D-dimers.
d. CT pulmonary angiogram.
e. Isotope lung scan.

†28 An 82-year-old female patient is receiving a blood transfusion on her first postoperative day following a right hemi-arthroplasty. Her baseline observations are normal. Five minutes after the blood transfusion is commenced her observations are as shown in Table 2.

Table 2. Results of observations.					
Pulse rate	**BP**	**Respiratory rate**		**SpO$_2$**	**Temp**
132 bpm	85/45mm Hg	16 bpm		97%	38.8°C

What is the most likely cause of her condition?

a. Postoperative chest infection.
b. Pyrexia of unknown origin.
c. Transfusion-related acute lung injury.
d. ABO incompatability.
e. Non-haemolytic febrile transfusion reaction.

29 A 72-year-old gentleman is scheduled for a total knee replacement. At the pre-operative assessment clinic, clinical examination reveals a small scar below the left clavicle. On questioning, the patient admits to having 'something' inserted in that area about 6 years ago. He has no particular symptoms and could not remember what the device was inserted for, but did confirm that it was checked to be in working condition in the clinic last month. No further documentation was available in the patient's notes. Which of the following is the most important next step in this patient's peri-operative management?

a. A plain chest radiograph should be performed to confirm the presence of a pacemaker.

b.   The pacemaker clinic should be contacted to confirm the indication
     for the pacemaker, type of pacemaker, and degree of pacemaker
     dependency.
c.   The diathermy plate should be placed as far as possible from the
     chest.
d.   A magnet should be placed over the pacemaker to ensure inhibition
     of shock therapy.
e.   Invasive blood pressure monitoring should be considered as an
     alternative to ECG monitoring.

30 A 26-year-old primigravida had an epidural for labour analgesia
    which was inserted uneventfully and remained *in situ* for 12 hours.
    Seven days postpartum the patient presented to the accident and
    emergency department with a low-grade fever, backache and
    weakness of the legs. The results of all routine blood investigations
    are within the normal range. The most likely diagnosis in this patient
    is:

a.   Epidural abscess.
b.   Intervertebral disc prolapse.
c.   Subdural haematoma.
d.   Obstetric palsy.
e.   Spinal arachnoiditis.

Set 5 answers

1   Answer: C. Fibromyalgia.

Fibromyalgia is characterised by chronic widespread pain and muscle tenderness. Other associated symptoms include fatigue, poor sleep, functional bowel disturbances, and joint stiffness. It is frequently associated with psychiatric conditions such as anxiety and depression.

The diagnosis of fibromyalgia is difficult as, in most cases, laboratory testing appears normal and many of the symptoms mimic those of other rheumatic conditions such as arthritis or osteoporosis. The most widely accepted criteria (stated by the American College of Rheumatology) for diagnosing fibromyalgia are a history of widespread pain lasting more than 3 months affecting both sides of body, above and below the waist, and the patient must feel pain at 11 or more tender points, of a designated 18 points on the surface of the body. Cognitive behavioural therapy (CBT), along with exercise, provides the greatest benefit in this group of patients.

In muscular dystrophy, there is progressive, symmetrical skeletal muscle weakness and wasting with intact sensation and reflexes. It is often associated with mental retardation.

Polymyalgia rheumatica is characterized by pain and stiffness in proximal muscles such as the pelvic and shoulder girdle, which is worse in the morning. Clinical examination usually demonstrates absence of tenderness and normal muscle strength. It is often associated with giant cell arthritis.

Further reading

1. Goldenberg DL. Multidisciplinary modalities in the treatment of fibromyalgia. *Journal of Clinical Psychiatry* 2008; 69: 30-4.
2. Nochimson G. Polymyalgia rheumatica. (http://emedicine.medscape.com/article/808755-overview).

2   Answer: C. Hypermagnesaemia.

Magnesium sulphate is used for seizure prophylaxis in severe pre-eclampsia and is often continued postpartum for several hours. This patient had features suggestive of hypermagnesaemia. The clinical features range from nausea and vomiting to respiratory and cardiac arrest, depending on the serum magnesium level. A marked reduction in tendon reflexes indicates impending magnesium toxicity. Monitoring should include the regular assessment of tendon reflexes. A marked depression of patellar reflexes is an indication of impending magnesium toxicity. The ECG may show a prolonged PR interval and intraventricular conduction defects. Respiratory rate, tendon reflexes and urine output should be monitored during magnesium therapy. If prolonged infusion or higher doses are used, serum magnesium levels should be monitored to prevent magnesium toxicity.

The classic ECG changes in pulmonary embolism include the S1Q3T3 pattern with a prominent S wave in lead I, and prominent Q and T waves in lead III. Amniotic fluid embolism usually occurs during labour, and can also occur during Caesarean section.

Further reading

1. Diseases associated with pregnancy. In: *Anesthesia and co-existing disease*, 4th ed. Stoelting RK, Dierdorf SF, Eds. Philadelphia, USA: Churchill Livingstone, 2002: 662.
2. Magnesium sulphate. In: *Analgesia, anaesthesia and preganancy, a practical guide.* Yentis SM, Grighouse D, May A, Bogod D, Elton C, Eds. London: W.B. Saunders, 2002: 198-200.
3. Novello NP, Blumstein HA. Hypermagnesemia. (http://emedicine.medscape.com/article/766604-overview).

3 Answer: B. Physostigmine.

Atropine has numerous side effects including dizziness, nausea, blurred vision, loss of balance, dilated pupils, photophobia, supraventricular or ventricular tachycardia, ventricular fibrillation, and, notably in the elderly, extreme confusion, dissociative hallucinations, and agitation. The CNS effects of atropine are due to its ability to cross the blood brain barrier, being a tertiary amine compound. The central anticholinergic symptoms are relatively common in the elderly. These symptoms range in severity from mild confusion to severe agitation, hallucinations, psychosis, seizures and coma ('anticholinergic syndrome'). Physostigmine is an anticholinesterase which crosses the blood brain barrier and therefore acts as an antidote to atropine. It is specifically indicated when the patient develops tachydysrhythmias with subsequent haemodynamic compromise, intractable seizures, severe agitation or psychosis.

Agitation and convulsions associated with anticholinergic toxicity can be controlled with intravenous midazolam, but physostigmine is the most specific antidote. Neostigmine does not cross the blood brain barrier and therefore is not useful in the treatment of anticholinergic syndrome.

Haloperidol is a member of the butyrophenone group of antipsychotic drugs used in the treatment of delirium, acute psychosis, and an adjunctive treatment during alcohol and opioid withdrawal.

Clonidine is a α2 agonist; it can be used as a supplement for sedation in intensive care for controlling agitation.

Further reading
1. Burns MJ, Linden CH, Graudins A, *et al.* A comparison of physostigmine and benzodiazepines for the treatment of anticholinergic poisoning. *Ann Emerg Med* 2000; 35: 374-81.

4 Answer: B. *Legionella pneumophilia.*

The most common pathogens causing community-acquired pneumonia (CAP) are *Streptococcus pneumoniae*, *Legionella pneumophilia* and

Staphylococcus aureus. A history of recent travel should be an alert to the possibility of *Legionella pneumophilia*, which is an aerobic gram negative bacillus. It is present in natural habitats such as fresh water ponds and lakes, and also reservoirs and artificial sources such as cooling towers and air conditioning systems. It is most commonly seen in younger patients and smokers. Patients may present with altered mental status, elevated liver enzymes, and diarrhoea, in addition to multilobar pneumonia.

Further reading
1. Sadashivaiah B, Carr B. Severe community-acquired pneumonia. *British Journal of Anaesthesia CEACCP* 2009; 9: 87-91.

5   Answer: A. Domperidone and ondansetron.

Parkinson's disease is a neurological condition involving the extrapyramidal system. It occurs due to loss of dopaminergic neurones in the substantia nigra, causing an imbalance of acetylcholine and dopamine. It is characterised by tremor, rigidity and postural instability. It is usually treated using dopamine precursors (e.g. levodopa), dopamine agonists (e.g. apomorphine), and MAO inhibitors (e.g. selegiline). Surgical treatment (deep brain stimulation) is reserved for those patients suffering from refractory disease with severe disablement.

Several drugs used during the peri-operative period may have an adverse effect on Parkinsonism. Opiates are often necessary after major surgery, but may worsen muscle rigidity. Pethidine should be avoided as it can cause hypertension and muscle rigidity in patients on selegiline. Patients may not be able to physically use patient-controlled analgesia (PCA). Antipsychotics, e.g. phenothiazines and butyrophenones, used as anti-emetics, may worsen symptoms of Parkinsonism, as they have antidopaminergic actions. Propofol may have dopamine-like effects, and thus helps to reduce tremor and muscle rigidity. Anticholinergic drugs which cross the blood brain barrier, such as atropine, can precipitate central anticholinergic syndrome. Glycopyrrolate is the anticholinergic of choice. Anti-emetics, such as metoclopramide, droperidol and prochlorperazine, may worsen the symptoms of Parkinsonism and cause extra-pyramidal effects. The anti-emetic of choice is domperidone as it does not cross the blood brain barrier and thus does not cause extra-pyramidal effects. 5-HT3 antagonists (e.g. ondansetron, granisetron) and cyclizine can safely be used.

Further reading
1. Nicholson G, Pereira AC, Hall GM. Parkinson's disease and anaesthesia. *British Journal of Anaesthesia* 2002; 89: 904-16.

6   Answer: C. Chemical lumbar sympathectomy.

Chemical sympatholysis is commonly performed for palmar or plantar hyperhidrosis, Buerger's disease, and critical lower limb ischaemia where there is no revascularization option available for palliative treatment of the pain.

The lumbar sympathetic chain lies on the anterolateral border of the vertebral body. The sympathetic chain is separated from the main lumbar sensory / motor nerves by the psoas muscle.

The block is performed using X-ray screening, intravenous sedation if necessary, and local anaesthetic infiltration, with the patient in the prone or lateral position. The needle is inserted about 8-10cm from the midline, and advanced so that it initially touches the side of the L2 or L3 vertebral body. It is then withdrawn slightly and readvanced until it slips past the anterolateral border of the vertebral body. Radio-opaque dye is injected to confirm the correct needle position. Complications include abdominal organ puncture, bleeding due to aortic and inferior vena cava injury, and genitofemoral neuralgia. Genitofemoral neuralgia is thought to be due to bruising of the L1 nerve root by the needle passing by it. More than 90% of cases recover spontaneously after 6 weeks. It is dangerous to perform the block in the presence of a large aortic aneurysm. Intravascular injection should be avoided by checking the needle tip position using a radio-opaque dye.

Lumbar epidural and nerve root blocks are useful for treatment of radicular pain in the legs but are not effective in ischaemic vascular pain. A superior hypogastric plexus block may be effective for the management of pelvic pain.

Further reading

1. Nesargikar P, Ajit M, Eyers P, *et al.* Lumbar chemical sympathectomy in peripheral vascular disease: does it still have a role? *International Journal of Surgery* 2009; 7: 145-9.

7 Answer: D. Needle decompression and insertion of a chest drain.

Pneumothorax is a recognised complication of laparoscopy. Gas passes from the peritoneum directly into the pleural space either through pre-existing channels, or it may spread from the mediastinum along the bronchi until it breaks through the weak spot into the pleural cavity. The distended neck veins (increased CVP), hypotension and desaturation suggest development of a tension pneumothorax. The specific treatment is needle decompression followed by insertion of a chest drain.

Increasing minute ventilation may improve the desaturation due to hypoventilation. An endotracheal tube blocked by a mucous plug can result in high airway pressures and desaturation which may be improved by endotracheal suction. PEEP is useful in improving oxygenation due to atelectasis.

Further reading

1. Farn J, Hammerman A, Brunt LM. Intraoperative pneumothorax during laparoscopic cholecystectomy: a complication of prior transdiaphragmatic surgery. *Surgical Laparoscopy Endoscopy & Percutaneous Techniques* 1993; 3: 219-22.
2. Complications and contraindications of laparoscopic surgery. In: *Anaesthesia for minimally invasive surgery.* Crozier TA, Ed. Cambridge: Cambridge University Press, 2004.

8 Answer: B. Small cell carcinoma of the lung.

The clinical features in this patient are suggestive of bronchial carcinoma. The syndrome of inappropriate ADH secretion (SIADH) from the posterior pituitary is a recognised manifestation of para-neoplastic syndrome associated with bronchial carcinoma (more commonly with small cell carcinoma). SIADH is one of the most common causes of hyponatraemia.

Other endocrine disorders associated with lung cancer include increased ACTH secretion, hyperparathyroidism and carcinoid syndrome.

Cerebral salt wasting syndrome causes hyponatraemia, and is seen in patients with traumatic brain injury. Both hypothyroidism and adrenal insufficiency can cause hyponatraemia but in this patient, the clinical history does not suggest these as a cause. SIADH secretion can also be associated with respiratory inflammatory diseases and infections such as tuberculosis, pneumonia, asthma and lung abscess.

149

Further reading

1. Craig S. Hyponatremia. (http://emedicine.medscape.com/article/767624-overview).
2. Reid PT, Innes JA. Respiratory disease. In: *Davidson's principles and practice of medicine*, 20th ed. Boon AN, Colledge NR, Walker BR, Hunter JAA, Eds. London: Churchill Livingstone, 2006; Chapter19: 705-11.
3. Ellison DH, Berl T. Clinical practice. The syndrome of inappropriate antidiuresis. *N Engl J Med* 2007; 356: 2064-72.

9 Answer: E. Guillain-Barré syndrome.

Guillain-Barré syndrome is an acute inflammatory demyelinating polyneuropathy affecting the peripheral nervous system. It is usually triggered by an acute infection. Most patients present with an acute neuropathy with ascending paralysis, hyporeflexia or areflexia, and raised protein concentrations in CSF.

Myasthenia gravis is an autoimmune disease affecting the neuromuscular system characterised by fluctuating muscle weakness commonly involving voluntary muscles, often the facial and eye muscles. The reflexes are not lost and the weakness generally improves with rest. The diagnosis can be confirmed by the edrophonium test.

Transverse myelitis is a neurological disorder caused by inflammation across both sides of one level, or segment, of the spinal cord. Symptoms of transverse myelitis include a loss of spinal cord function occurring over several hours to several weeks. It usually begins as a sudden onset of lower back pain, muscle weakness, or abnormal sensations in the toes and feet, and can rapidly progress to more severe symptoms, including paralysis, urinary retention, and loss of bowel control. Bladder and bowel dysfunction is common. Many patients also report muscle spasms, a general feeling of discomfort, headache, fever, and loss of appetite. Pain is the primary presenting symptom of transverse myelitis in approximately one third to one half of all patients. Severe electrolyte disturbances can cause generalised muscle weakness. EMG and neurological studies are normal.

Motor neurone disease (MND) is a progressive neurodegenerative disease that attacks the upper and lower motor neurones. Degeneration of the motor neurones leads to weakness and wasting of muscles, causing increasing loss of mobility in the limbs, and difficulties with speech, swallowing and breathing.

Further reading

1. Hughes RAC, Cornblath DR. Guillain-Barré syndrome. *Lancet* 2005; 366: 1653-66.

10   Answer: C. Subarachnoid block.

Complications of cervical plexus block include subarachnoid block, epidural block, intravascular injection resulting in local anaesthetic toxicity, phrenic nerve palsy, recurrent laryngeal nerve palsy, Horner's syndrome, haematoma and airway obstruction. Subarachnoid block may also occur during retrobulbar block, interscalene brachial plexus block and stellate ganglion block.

Epidural block is a possible complication but it is slower in onset and unlikely to produce profound hypotension. Accidental intravenous injection of local anaesthetic agent may result in local anaesthetic toxicity. The clinical features of local anaesthteic toxicity include tinnitus, circumoral numbness, seizures, respiratory depression, apnoea, bradycardia, conduction abnormalities and hypotension. As this patient recovered rapidly, this is unlikely to be local anaesthetic toxicity. Phrenic nerve palsy may result in shortness of breath due to diaphragmatic weakness.

Further reading

1. Carling A, Simmonds M. Complications from regional anaesthesia for carotid endarterectomy. *British Journal of Anaesthesia* 2000; 84: 797-800.
2. Ross S, Scarborough CD. Total spinal anaesthesia following brachial plexus block. *Anesthesiology* 1973; 39: 458.
3. Edde RR, Deutsch S. Cardiac arrest after interscalene brachial plexus block. *Anesthesia Analgesia* 1977; 56: 446-7.

11 Answer: C. Sub-Tenon's block.

Anaesthesia for cataract surgery can be provided using local and general techniques. Local anaesthetic techniques can be divided into superficial eye blocks such as sub-Tenon's, or topical anaesthesia alone, and deep eye blocks via the peribulbar and retrobulbar routes.

Prophylactic anticoagulation is common in patients presenting for cataract surgery, and there may be significant risks arising from cessation of such therapy. Topical anaesthesia or sub-Tenon's block can be safely used in the anticoagulated patient. Since this patient has COAD, it would be wise to avoid a general anaesthetic. With peribulbar and retrobulbar blocks the risk of retrobulbar haemorrhage is quite significant. Patients with myopia are likely to have an axial length of more than 25mm and are at risk of globe perforation during retrobulbar block.

Further reading

1. Kumar C, Dodds C. Ophthalmic regional block. *Ann Acad Med Singapore* 2006; 35: 158-67.

12 Answer: D. Isoprenaline.

The transplanted heart does not receive autonomic input because it is denervated during harvesting. It does not respond to extrinsic neural signals although intrinsic myocardial mechanisms and reflexes are intact. It responds to circulating catecholamines and directly acting sympathomimetic agents. Vagolytic drugs such as atropine and glycopyrrolate will not increase the heart rate. Ephedrine and norephedrine are indirectly-acting sympathomimetic drugs and do not have any response on the denervated heart. Isoprenaline is a potent synthetic directly-acting catecholamine. It stimulates both $\beta1$ and $\beta2$ receptors. It increases the heart rate, myocardial contractility and cardiac output.

Further reading

1. Stone ME. Non-cardiac surgery after heart transplantation. In: *Clinical cases in anaesthesia*, 3rd ed. Reed AP, Yudkowitz FS, Eds. Philadelphia, USA: Elsevier Churchill Livingstone, 2005; Case 12: 59-64.

13 Answer: B. Giant unilateral lung cyst.

Absolute indications for lung isolation include a giant unilateral lung cyst or bulla, broncho-pleural fistula, open surgery on the main bronchus, unilateral massive haemorrhage and infection in one of the lungs where contamination of the other lung is to be avoided. The use of a double-lumen tube facilitates the ventilation of the normal lung in conditions such as a unilateral lung cyst and bulla, thereby avoiding barotrauma. Relative indications for lung isolation include lobectomy, thoracic spinal surgery, thoracic aneurysm repair and pneumonectomy.

Further reading

1. Eastwood J, Mahajan R. One lung anaesthesia. *British Journal of Anaesthesia CEACCP* 2002; 2: 83-7.

14   Answer: D. Nitroglycerine and dobutamine.

The clinical picture is suggestive of pulmonary hypertension. The ideal drug combination in this patient is one which increases myocardial contractility, and decreases the pulmonary and systemic vascular resistance. A combination of dobutamine and nitroglycerine would be the most suitable. Dobutamine has agonist action on β1 receptors, acts as a positive inotrope and therefore increases the cardiac output. Nitroglycerine reduces pulmonary vascular resistance and systemic vascular resistance and thereby reduces pulmonary congestion and augments cardiac output. Noradrenaline will increase the systemic vascular resistance and may worsen the pulmonary congestion. Propranolol will further increase the pulmonary vascular resistance by its β-antagonist action and also will reduce cardiac contractility.

Further reading

1.   Rudarakanchana N, Trembath RC, Morrell NW. New insights into the pathogenesis and treatment of primary pulmonary hypertension. *Thorax* 2001; 56: 888-90.

15   Answer: B. Transoesophageal echocardiography.

The ECG is most commonly used to detect intra-operative ischaemia and rhythm disturbances but the ST segment analysis on standard monitors has poor sensitivity and specificity. Transoesophageal echocardiography is the most sensitive monitor for detection of myocardial ischaemia. It demonstrates regional wall motion abnormalities, an early sign of myocardial ischaemia. These changes are seen before the ECG changes develop. Pulmonary artery diastolic pressures increase during myocardial ischaemia. Dipyridamole-thallium scanning may be used to detect peri-operative myocardial perfusion defects. There are, however, limited data on the use of this technique during the intra-operative period.

Further reading

1.   Shore-Lesserson LJ. Coronary artery bypass grafting. In: *Clinical cases in anaesthesia*, 3rd ed. Reed AP, Yudkowitz FS, Eds. Philadelphia, USA: Elsevier Churchill Livingstone, 2005; Case 13: 65-8.

2. Edwards ND, Reilly CS. Detection of peri-operative myocardial ischaemia, review article. *British Journal of Anaesthesia* 1994; 72: 104-15.

16   Answer: D. Lidocaine 5% plasters.

The clinical presentation of this patient's pain, her age, and recent course of steroids, all indicate that she is suffering from post-herpetic neuralgia (PHN). The reactivation of the *Herpes zoster* virus occurs due to immunosuppression and therefore is more commonly seen in patients with old age, poor nutrition, malignancy, and immunosuppression due to any cause. PHN is treated using lidocaine 5% plasters, tricyclic antidepressants (amitriptyline), calcium channel blockers (gabapentin, pregabalin), sodium channel blockers (phenytoin and carbamazepine) and non-pharmacological therapies such as TENS, acupuncture and cognitive behavioural therapy (CBT). In this particular patient, lidocaine 5% plasters would be most appropriate. The soothing effect of the plaster will minimise the pain from mechanical allodynia and will also provide local analgesia without any systemic side effects. This patient has multiple comorbidities so it would be wise to avoid any systemic therapy.

Further reading

1. Guy H, *et al.* Efficacy and tolerability of a 5% lidocaine medicated plaster for the topical treatment of post-herpetic neuralgia: results of a long-term study. *Current Medical Research and Opinion* 2009; 25: 1295-305.

17   Answer: D. Ruptured valve cusp of the mitral valve.

Infective bacterial endocarditis is most commonly observed in adults, but the incidence in children with congenital heart disease or central indwelling venous catheters continues to rise.

Patients with acute bacterial endocarditis present with an acute, toxic, febrile illness and symptoms that have lasted less than 2 weeks. There may be a history of intravenous drug use. *Staphylococcus aureus* is the most common cause of acute bacterial endocarditis. Patients with subacute bacterial endocarditis present with more non-specific flu-like symptoms that have lasted more than 2 weeks. Subacute bacterial endocarditis is more common in patients with an underlying congenital heart defect, a bicuspid aortic valve being the most common example. *Staphylococcus aureus* is the primary organism causing endocarditis. Other organisms include *Streptococcus viridans*, *Streptococcus intermedius* and *Pseudomonas aeruginosa*.

Acute heart failure may occur due to valve destruction or distortion and/or rupture of the chordae tendinae. Chronic heart failure may be due to progressive valvular insufficiency with worsening ventricular function. Heart failure with aortic insufficiency is associated with a high mortality rate.

Further reading
1. Bayer AS, Bolger AF, Taubert KA, *et al.* Diagnosis and management of infective endocarditis and its complications. *Circulation* 1998; 98: 2936-48.

18 Answer: A. Rapid sequence induction, intubation and commencement of positive pressure ventilation.

The clinical information along with the raised respiratory rate and low PaO_2 suggests the diagnosis of acute life-threatening asthma. Appropriate first-line treatment has already been started, but there are no signs of a response.

There is little good quality evidence regarding drug therapy for the further management of severe asthma. The use of aminophylline is limited due to its side effects (arrhythmias, restlessness, vomiting, and convulsions), related to a narrow therapeutic window. Intravenous salbutamol has no benefit compared to nebulised salbutamol provided administration of nebulisers is not a problem. In practice this means that intravenous β2 agonists should generally be reserved for patients who are ventilated.

There is some evidence that magnesium sulphate may be of benefit in severe asthma, and importantly has few side effects when given as a single dose. Although further research is undoubtedly required, the best supporting evidence for all second-line agents suggests the use of magnesium.

Intubation and ventilation of patients with severe asthma is difficult and can have deleterious effects both at the time of intubation and during mechanical ventilation. It should be used in the presence of life-threatening hypoxia, cardiac or respiratory arrest or after all other medical treatment has failed.

Heliox (79% helium and 21% oxygen) will reduce the work of breathing in acute upper airway obstruction by improving the turbulent flow due to low density of helium. It has been suggested in severe asthma but it limits the FiO_2 that can be achieved and has no role in acute life-threatening asthma.

Further reading
1. British guideline in the management of asthma. British Thoracic Society, 2009.
2. Stanley D, Tunnicliffe W. Management of life-threatening asthma in adults. *British Journal of Anaesthesia CEACCP* 2008; 8: 95-9.

19 Answer: A. Intravenous infusion of mannitol 0.5g/kg.

Mannitol is an osmotic diuretic that reduces ICP by drawing fluid from the brain. It has been shown to improve surgical access and reduce ICP within a few minutes of administration. It can also temporarily improve cerebral perfusion by increasing intra-vascular volume.

Hyperventilation is a recognised method of reducing ICP as cerebral blood flow follows an almost linear relationship with $PaCO_2$. However, hyperventilation to sub-normal levels of CO_2 can cause significant vasoconstriction and has the potential to cause ischaemia in vulnerable brain tissue. The $PaCO_2$ should be maintained >4.0kPa unless other methods of reducing ICP have failed.

Steroids have no role in reducing ICP in acute head injury; they are only useful in reducing the bulk of tumours and intracranial infective lesions. A large-scale study has found evidence of increased mortality with the administration of steroids in acute head injury.

Hypertension and hypervolaemia are important in order to maintain cerebral perfusion in the presence of cerebral vasospasm, but other treatments will be needed to reduce intracranial pressure.

Further reading
1. Mishra LD, Rajkumar N, Hancock SM. Current controversies in neuroanaesthesia, head injury management and neurocritical care. *British Journal of Anaesthesia CEACCP* 2006; 6: 79-82.

20 Answer: D. Infiltration of 5ml 0.5% levobupivacaine at the elbow between the brachioradialis and the biceps tendon.

In this case the axillary nerve block has spared part of the radial nerve distribution. The patient is very keen to have surgery performed under a regional block so general anaesthesia should be used only if other measures fail.

Repeating the axillary block has a high chance of being successful, although response to nerve stimulation will be unreliable; this could be performed under ultrasound guidance. However, by performing the block again with the same amount of levobupivacaine, the total dose will exceed the maximum safe dose.

Nerve blocks at the elbow, while unlikely to provide adequate anaesthesia alone, are useful to supplement a problematic brachial plexus block. Blocking the radial nerve at the elbow will most likely resolve the problem and allow the procedure to be performed.

21 Answer: D. Spinal cord stimulation.

This patient is suffering from failed back surgery syndrome (post-laminectomy syndrome). This manifests as a combination of chronic neuropathic and nociceptive pain mainly involving the legs and/or the lower back following successful spinal surgery. This patient's history suggests minimal psycho-social issues and therefore spinal cord stimulation would be the most appropriate next step in his treatment. A spinal cord stimulator (SCS) provides pulsed electrical signals to the spinal cord to relieve pain from various conditions. In the simplest form, it consists of stimulating electrodes implanted in the extradural space, an implanted electrical pulse generator, wires connecting the electrodes to the generator, and the generator remote control.

Electrotherapy of pain by neurostimulation was first used shortly after proposal of the gate control theory. The theory proposed that nerves carrying painful peripheral stimuli and nerves carrying touch and vibratory sensation both terminate in the dorsal horn (the gate) of the spinal cord. It was hypothesized that input to the latter could be manipulated in order to 'close' the gate. The mechanisms of action of spinal cord stimulation in relieving neuropathic pain may be very different from that involving ischaemic pain. In neuropathic pain, evidence shows that SCS alters the local neurochemistry in the dorsal horn, suppressing the hyper-excitability of the neurones. There is some evidence that there are increased levels of serotonin and GABA, and suppressed levels of excitatory amino acids such as glutamate. In the case of ischaemic pain, analgesia seems to be mediated by inhibition of the sympathetic nervous system and vasodilatation. SCS is used mostly in the treatment of radicular pain in the lower limb (failed back surgery syndrome), complex regional pain syndrome affecting the limbs, and ischaemic pain (e.g. ischaemic leg pain, refractory angina).

Further reading
1. Oakley J, Prager J. Spinal cord stimulation: mechanism of action. *Spine* 2002; 27: 2574-83.

22 Answer: C. Stroke volume variation of 12%.

Although central venous pressure (CVP) is widely used for assessing fluid status, in reality it is a poor guide. A single reading of CVP bears little relationship to the right ventricular end-diastolic volume, and as such does not measure the degree of filling. The same is true of the pulmonary capillary occlusion pressure as an assessment of left ventricular filling. These non-linear relationships are thought to be due to dynamic changes in ventricular wall compliance.

A low urine output may be suggestive of hypovolaemia, but on its own is not diagnostic. There are several other possible causes of acute renal failure in the sick surgical patient. Equally, prolonged capillary refill time represents poor peripheral perfusion, but this is not necessarily due to hypovolaemic shock.

Stroke volume variation can be measured by pulse contour analysis or by Doppler ultrasound of the aorta. In clinical trials a stroke volume variation of >9.5% has been shown to be highly predictive of a response to a fluid bolus.

Further reading
1. Eyre L, Breen A. Optimal volaemic status and predicting fluid responsiveness. *British Journal of Anaesthesia CEACCP* 2010; 10: 59-62.

23 Answer: B. Stop the epidural infusion and reassess after 2 hours.

The differential diagnosis in this case includes excessive administration of an epidural local anaesthetic, an epidural abscess and an epidural haematoma. The latter two are serious complications and must be acted upon as soon as they are diagnosed. They are, however, much less likely than an excessive block so this should be ruled out first. It would be appropriate to stop the infusion first and reassess within a fairly short time period. If there is no sign of the block receding then an immediate imaging and neurosurgical referral should be arranged.

A normal temperature makes an abscess unlikely, although it cannot be ruled out. It would also be unlikely for an abscess to form this soon after insertion. It is unnecessary to start antibiotics without objective evidence of abscess formation. Equally, the facts in this case do not entirely support the diagnosis of an epidural haematoma; a prophylactic dose of low-molecular-weight heparin is unlikely to cause haematoma formation and the INR of 1.1 is within the normal range. There is no indication for the administration of blood products or clotting factors in this case.

Further reading
1. Grewal S, Hocking G, Wildsmith JA. Epidural abscesses. *British Journal of Anaesthesia* 2006; 96: 292-302.

24   Answer: A. Lorazepam 4mg I.V.

The clinical features and history of drug abuse, and the intake of citalopram suggests serotonin syndrome. This is characterised by the triad of altered level of consciousness, neuromuscular hyperactivity and autonomic instability. The treatment is mainly supportive and should follow an ABC approach. Benzodiazepines or phenytoin are used for the management of convulsions. Activated charcoal is useful but only within the first hour. Cyproheptadine and chlorpromazine have been used but there is no evidence to support their use. Alkalinization of urine is useful in reducing the incidence of renal failure.

Further reading
1. Ward W, Sair M. Oral poisoning: an update. *British Journal of Anaesthesia CEACCP* 2010; 10: 6-11.

25   Answer: D. 10ml/kg of 0.9% saline.

This child has severe diabetic ketoacidosis (DKA) with signs of marked intravascular fluid depletion (severe tachycardia, hypotension and raised lactate). A cautious 10ml/kg fluid bolus should be given (10-20ml/kg 0.9% saline over the first 1-2 hours) and the response assessed. Hypotonic fluids should not be used. Children with DKA are at high risk of developing cerebral oedema. DKA results in low 2,3-diphosphoglycerate (2,3 DPG), which reduces the oxygen delivery to the tissues. This effect of low 2,3 DPG is opposed by a low pH which shifts the oxygen dissociation curve to the right. Intravenous bicarbonate shifts the oxygen dissociation curve to the left, and along with low 2,3 DPG it reduces the oxygen delivery to the tissues. Hypertonic saline or mannitol should be given if cerebral oedema is suspected. Insulin is best administered as a low dose I.V. infusion rather than a bolus dose. A low-dose infusion of 0.1unit/kg/hour should achieve an adequate steady state plasma level within an hour. An I.V. bolus dose may increase the risk of cerebral oedema.

Further reading
1. Steel S, Tibby SM. Paediatric diabetic ketoacidosis. *British Journal of Anaesthesia CEACCP* 2009; 9: 194-9.

26 Answer: E. Enoxaparin 1mg/kg subcutaneously every 12 hours.

DVT carries considerable clinical risk during pregnancy, and treatment should be started prior to the Doppler scan if the diagnosis has been made on clinical grounds. Warfarin should be avoided during pregnancy due to the risk of teratogenicity. As the clearance of heparin is increased during pregnancy, the dose of enoxaparin in pregnancy is raised to 1.0mg/kg twice daily. Monitoring should include anti-Xa activity (target 0.6-1.0 units/ml) and platelet count. Administration of enoxaparin should cease once labour begins. The duration of treatment should normally be 6 months, but if started early in pregnancy then enoxaparin should continue at the full treatment dose until 6 weeks post-delivery.

Further reading
1. Thromboembolic disease in pregnancy and the puerperium. Guidelines and Audit Committee of RCOG, April 2001.

27 Answer: B. Echocardiography.

This patient has risk factors for and clinical features of a massive pulmonary embolism (PE). Because of her haemodynamic compromise a bedside echocardiogram would be the test of choice to confirm diagnosis prior to consideration of thrombolytic therapy. A CT pulmonary angiogram would be the initial investigation in a stable patient. D-dimers are only recommended in patients with a low to intermediate clinical risk of PE. Isotope lung scanning may be considered in stable patients with a normal chest X-ray and no concurrent cardiopulmonary disease. Troponin may rise and be a prognostic indicator but is not diagnostic.

Further reading
1. van Beek EJR, Elliot CA, Kiely DG. Diagnosis and initial treatment of patients with suspected pulmonary embolism. *British Journal of Anaesthesia CEACCP* 2009; 4: 119-24.
2. British Thoracic Society guidelines for the management of suspected pulmonary embolism. *Thorax* 2003; 58: 470-83.

28 Answer: D. ABO incompatability.

This patient did not have respiratory distress or hypoxaemia; this makes postoperative chest infection and transfusion-related acute lung injury unlikely causes for this clinical presentation. A non-haemolytic febrile transfusion reaction can develop up to several hours afterwards but is more common around 30 minutes into the transfusion. It is very common and only rarely leads to more severe symptoms such as hypotension, vomiting and respiratory distress. ABO incompatability should be suspected when the symptoms occur within a few minutes of commencing transfusion. It is important that the diagnosis is made rapidly so that transfusion is stopped immediately and supportive management is commenced promptly.

Further reading
1. Serious Hazards of Transfusion Annual Report 2008.
2. Maxwell MJ, Wilson MJA. Complications of blood transfusion. *British Journal of Anaesthesia CEACCP* 2006; 6: 225-9.
3. Blood transfusion and the anaesthetist. Red cell transfusion 2. AAGBI guidelines, 2008.
4. British Committee for Standards in Haematology (BSCH). Guidelines for administration of blood and blood components and the management of transfused patients. *Transfusion Medicine* 1999; 9: 227-38.

29 Answer: B. The pacemaker clinic should be contacted to confirm the indication for the pacemaker, type of pacemaker, and degree of pacemaker dependency.

In all planned surgical procedures, both the anaesthetist and the surgeon should be made aware of the presence of a pacemaker. In this instance, the patient is unable to give the indication for the use of the pacemaker nor the device type; therefore, the pacemaker clinic should be contacted for more clinical information. A chest X-ray will give some device information but would not confirm whether the device has been checked recently. Interference from monopolar diathermy remains a risk even if the operative site is far from the pacemaker and this mode should only be used as a last resort. Bipolar diathermy should be used whenever possible but interference is still possible. A magnet will in many cases inhibit delivery of shock therapy but this is not guaranteed and may vary between manufacturers. In the presence of electromagnetic interference (EMI), the magnet may alter the programmability of the pacemaker, resulting in malfunction. Its use is not indicated for programmable pacemakers. In addition to an ECG, an alternative method of monitoring heart rate should be considered in the presence of pacemaker spikes on the ECG.

Further reading
1. Guidelines for perioperative management of patients with implantable pacemakers or implantable cardioverter defibrillators. (http://www.mhra.gov.uk/Safetyinformation/General safety information and advice).

30 Answer: A. Epidural abscess.

The classical presentation of an epidural abscess is a triad of fever, backache and neurological deficit. Other signs or symptoms are epidural site redness, tenderness and purulent discharge at the site of insertion. Though these are the common symptoms, patients may present with just one or two of the above symptoms, hence, a high index of suspicion is necessary. The most common organism causing an epidural abscess is *Staphylococcus aureus*, which tracks from the skin along the catheter site.

The symptoms of intevertebral disc prolapse can vary depending on the location and severity. It can range from no pain to severe pain, radiating to regions supplied by the affected nerve root. Other symptoms may include sensory changes such as numbness, tingling, muscular weakness, and paralysis and sphincter disturbances. The presence of fever should raise suspicion of an epidural infection.

A subdural haematoma usually develops soon after the insertion of the epidural or after removal of the catheter. Symptoms begin with local or radicular back pain and compression of lumbar spinal roots may cause cauda equina syndrome. Neurological deficit progresses over minutes to hours.

Obstetric palsy can result in unilateral foot drop due to compression of the lumbosacral plexus by the large foetus or by forceps-assisted delivery. Maternal obstetric palsy is a common transient weakness in the distribution of nerves anywhere along the lumbosacral plexus. The condition can present commonly as meralgia paraesthetica (neuropathy of the lateral femoral cutaneous nerve), femoral neuropathy or sacral numbness. It occurs during the immediate postpartum period and gradually improves over a period of weeks.

Local inflammation of the arachnoid mater resulting in fibrosis, adhesions and scarring is known as arachnoiditis. The presence of blood in the subarachnoid space due to traumatic puncture, a high concentration of local anaesthetic (2% lidocaine, 0.75% bupivacaine), steroid injection and the preservatives in local anaesthetics, such as methyl-paraben or prophyl-paraben, can cause arachnoiditis. Usually the patient presents several weeks to months after the procedure with a neurological deficit in the lower extremity.

Further reading

1. Green LK, Paech MJ. Obstetric epidural catheter-related infections at a major teaching hospital: a retrospective case series. *International Journal of Obstetric Anaesthesia* 2010; 19: 38-43.
2. Sghirlanzoni A, Marrazzi R, Pareyson R, *et al.* Epidural anaesthesia and spinal arachnoiditis. *Anaesthesia* 1989; 44: 317-21.
3. Aldrete JA. Neurological deficit and arachnoiditis following neuroaxial anaesthesia. *Acta Anaesthesiol Scand* 2003; 47: 3-12.

Set 6 questions

1   A 42-year-old female is being seen in the pre-operative assessment clinic prior to an elective laparoscopic cholecystectomy. She gives a history of shortness of breath and fatigue on minimal exertion. Cardiovascular examination reveals a heart rate of 62 bpm, BP of 110/70mmHg and a mid-diastolic murmur. A postero-anterior view of the chest X-ray shows straightening of the left heart border. What is the most likely diagnosis?

a.   Mitral stenosis.
b.   Tricuspid stenosis.
c.   Mitral regurgitation.
d.   Aortic stenosis.
e.   Pulmonary stenosis.

2   A previously fit and well 2-year-old boy, weighing 12kg, presents to the emergency department with convulsions. He has been febrile and irritable during the day and started to fit in the evening, and an ambulance was called. Diazepam 6mg and paraldehyde 4.8ml were given rectally en route to hospital by the paramedics. His temperature is 38°C, and his SpO_2, BP and blood glucose are within normal limits. He is breathing spontaneously and maintaining his airway, and is receiving high-flow oxygen. Despite the above measures he has been fitting continuously for the last 20 minutes. You have managed to secure venous access. Which of the below would be the most appropriate medication to be given next?

a. Oral diazepam 0.5mg/kg.
b. Oral midazolam 0.5mg/kg.
c. Intravenous phenytoin 18mg/kg, given over 30 minutes.
d. Rapid sequence induction with thiopentone and suxamethonium.
e. Oral paracetamol 240mg.

3   You are called to the emergency department to assess a 35-year-old man who has been admitted with a suspected drug overdose. On examination, he appears confused and agitated and unable to give a clear history. His temperature is 38.6°C, pulse rate is 120 bpm, BP is 143/87mm Hg, respiratory rate is 18/minute and SpO$_2$ is 97% in room air. He also has a tremor, muscle weakness and hyper-reflexia. Assuming the diagnosis of overdose is correct, which of the following medications is most likely to be responsible for his symptoms?

a. Aspirin.
b. Lorazepam.
c. Edrophonium.
d. Citalopram.
e. Amitriptyline.

4   A 27-year-old man has been sedated and ventilated in the intensive care unit, following a head injury. Five days after admission it is noticed that his serum sodium concentration has dropped to 125mmol/L. Further tests reveal a haemoglobin concentration of 15g/dL, a haematocrit of 44% and a urea of 14mmol/L. Plasma and urine osmolarities are 295 and 600mosm/L, respectively. On clinical examination he appears dehydrated and it is noticed that his vasopressor requirements have increased. Which of the following is the most appropriate treatment for this problem?

a. Fluid restriction to 1L/24hours.
b. Titrated doses of intravenous desmopressin.
c. Intravenous infusion of 0.9% saline solution.
d. Administration of furosemide 20mg intravenously.
e. Demeclocycline 900mg daily.

5 A 46-year-old woman is due to have an elective total abdominal hysterectomy and oopherectomy for stage one endometrial cancer. General anaesthesia with a transversus abdominis plane block and postoperative patient-controlled analgesia have been planned. Which of the following would be the best means of providing venous thrombo-embolism (VTE) prophylaxis?

a. Anti-embolism stockings alone.
b. Mechanical VTE prophylaxis using a combination of anti-embolism stockings and an intermittent pneumatic device.
c. Mechanical VTE prophylaxis and low-molecular-weight heparin for 3 days post-surgery.
d. Mechanical VTE prophylaxis and low-molecular-weight heparin continued for 28 days post-surgery.
e. Low-molecular-weight heparin alone.

6 A 39-year-old patient, who has a 2-year history of opioid addiction, has had a below-knee amputation following a road traffic accident. On the third postoperative day, despite initial satisfactory pain control, he starts to suffer from severe increasing generalized stump pain. Increasing morphine dosage has been ineffective. Which one of the following analgesic regimes is the most likely to be effective in relieving his pain?

a. Epidural morphine infusion.
b. Intrathecal morphine infusion.
c. Intravenous ketamine infusion.
d. Intravenous morphine infusion.
e. Intravenous gabapentin infusion.

7 A 3-year-old boy known to be diabetic presents with irritability and disorientation. His blood glucose is 12mmol/L and his urine is positive for ketones. Which of the following is the most common cause of death in a patient presenting with these clinical features?

a. Sepsis.
b. Cerebral oedema.
c. Arrhythmias.
d. Acute pancreatitis.
e. Hypokalaemia.

8

A 45-year-old female patient is scheduled for arthroscopy of the shoulder joint. During pre-operative assessment, she gives a history of cold intolerance and weight gain. On examination her heart rate is 58 per minute and blood pressure is 130/72mmHg. Her blood test reveals an elevated TSH level and low T3 and T4 levels. Which of the following is the most likely cause for her symptoms?

a. Pituitary failure.
b. Hypothalamic failure.
c. Iodine deficiency.
d. Autoimmune hypothyroidism.
e. Hypophysectomy.

9

A 21-year-old university student has been admitted to the intensive care unit with a diagnosis of meningitis. He has no significant past medical history and presents with acute confusion after onset of a severe headache. He has been sedated and intubated because he became extremely agitated on arrival to the emergency department. A CT scan of the head is normal and the results of lumbar puncture are shown in Table 1.

Table 1. Results of lumbar puncture.

Neutrophils	Lymphocytes	Protein	Glucose
10/mm³	300/mm³	0.35g/L	5.9mmol/L

Which of the following organisms is most likely to have caused the meningitis?

a.   *Neisseria meningitidis.*
b.   *Streptococcus pneumoniae.*
c.   *Haemophilus influenzae* type B.
d.   *Myobacterium tuberculous.*
e.   *Herpes simplex* virus.

10 A 23-year-old male is admitted to the accident and emergency department following a motorcycle accident. He is found to have a GCS of 9/15. He is sedated, intubated and ventilated, and an urgent CT scan is performed. Which of the following findings in the CT scan would indicate the worst prognosis in the first 14 days?

a.   Subarachnoid bleed.
b.   Subdural haematoma.
c.   Depressed skull fracture.
d.   Obliteration of the third ventricle.
e.   An extradural haematoma.

11 You are assessing a new patient in the pain clinic. He is a 49-year-old patient who had an amputation of the right upper limb at the mid-humeral level 3 years ago. He is complaining of pain in the right wrist, which is associated with burning and a spasmodic sensation. What would be the most appropriate initial therapy for him?

a.   Morphine sulphate.
b.   Cognitive behavioural therapy.
c.   Image-guided physiotherapy.
d.   Gabapentin.
e.   Stellate ganglion block.

12 A 23-year-old male undergoes a closed reduction of a fracture of his right femur. In the immediate postoperative period he becomes tachypneoic and confused. Which of the following findings most strongly suggest fat embolism?

a. Axillary petechiae.
b. Emboli present in the retina.
c. Fat present in urine.
d. Fat globules present in the sputum.
e. Increasing ESR.

13 A 12-year-old girl with a history of cerebral palsy underwent insertion of a cochlear implant into the right ear under general anaesthesia. She had not received her morning dose of regular medications. The procedure took 3 hours with no adverse events during the intra-operative period and recovery. On return to the ward she experienced nausea and one episode of vomiting. About 6 hours later she became very disorientated and developed dystonia and painful muscle spasms. Which of the following regular medications would be the most likely to lead to these clinical features?

a. Ondansetron.
b. Diazepam.
c. Ibuprofen.
d. Sodium valproate.
e. Baclofen.

14 A 18-year-old female presents to the accident and emergency department having taken about 50 tablets of paracetamol. She says that she swallowed the tablets within the last 20 minutes. Which of the following treatments would be the most effective in reducing absorption of paracetamol?

a. Induced emesis.
b. Gastric lavage.
c. Activated charcoal.
d. N-acetyl cysteine.
e. Methionine.

15 A 24-year-old African man is scheduled for an urgent appendicectomy. His blood results and observations during pre-operative assessment are shown in Table 2.

Table 2. Observations and results of blood testing.			
Observations			
Heart rate	**BP**	**Temperature**	**SpO$_2$**
120 bpm	106/56mm Hg	38.2°C	95%
Blood results			
Hb	**WCC**	**Urea**	**Creatinine**
7.3g/dL	16.0	8.9mmol/L	143μmol/L

The most appropriate immediate management is:

a.   Laparotomy.
b.   Oxygen and intravenous Hartmann's solution.
c.   Sickledex testing.
d.   Blood transfusion to achieve Hb >10g/dl.
e.   Pre-optimisation in the anaesthetic room.

16 A 6-year-old child weighing 20kg is scheduled on a day-surgery list for circumcision. He is mildly asthmatic and has had ibuprofen in the past. His mother is quite worried about the postoperative pain. Which one of the following is most likely to provide adequate pain relief safely?

a.   Caudal block using 10ml of 0.5% bupivacaine.
b.   Penile block and regular paracetamol and ibuprofen.
c.   Regular ibuprofen and 4-hourly Oramorph for the first 24 hours.
d.   Regular paracetamol and 4-hourly Oramorph for the first 24 hours.
e.   Caudal block using 0.125% bupivacaine and ketamine 2mg/kg.

17 A 32-year-old female is scheduled for a laparoscopic cholecystectomy. Her medical history includes long QT syndrome which is treated with bisoprolol 5mg per day. In the past she suffered a cardiac arrest and now has a history of recurrent syncope. Which of the following should be the next step in her pre-operative management?

a. Increasing the dose of bisoprolol.
b. Antibradycardia pacing.
c. Intravenous magnesium sulphate 2g.
d. Insertion of an automatic implantable cardioverter defibrillator (AICD).
e. Oral amiodarone 300mg per day.

18 A 60-year-old ASA1 male patient is undergoing a radical prostatectomy under general anaesthesia. During the procedure the estimated total blood loss is 2L. He receives 4 units of blood and 4 units of fresh frozen plasma over a period of 30 minutes. About 2 hours following the blood transfusion, the patient develops tachycardia and hypotension requiring inotropic support with an epinephrine infusion. The peak airway pressure increases from 15 to 35cm H_2O. Clinical examination reveals bilateral lung crepitations. The most likely cause for his clinical deterioration is:

a. Sepsis.
b. Volume overload.
c. Myocardial infarction.
d. Transfusion-related acute lung injury (TRALI).
e. Cardiogenic shock.

19 A 62-year-old man collapses on the third postoperative day after undergoing an oesophagectomy. His medical history includes hypertension, angina, chronic smoking, and type II diabetes. His vital parameters after collapse are shown in Table 3.

Table 3. Vital parameters.			
Temperature	**BP**	**Pulse rate**	**CVP**
39.2°C	82/30mm Hg	114 bpm	2mmHg

Which of the following is the most likely cause of this clinical presentation?

a. Septicaemia.
b. Myocardial infarction.
c. Severe dehydration.
d. Haemorrhage.
e. Cardiac tamponade.

20 A 35-year-old male patient is scheduled for a laparoscopic cholecystectomy. He gives a history of muscular weakness affecting his breathing. He also has a history of obstructive sleep apnoea. Clinical examination reveals frontal baldness, ptosis and an inability to relax his hand grip. His muscle tone is increased significantly by exercise and cold. Which of the following pre-operative investigations would be the most important one to perform given this patient's condition?

a. Serum electrolytes.
b. Haemoglobin.
c. Ultrasound of his gall bladder.
d. Electromyography.
e. ECG.

21

A 6-week-old baby boy is admitted to hospital with projectile vomiting. Pyloric stenosis is diagnosed and he is scheduled for pyloromyotomy. He was born 2 weeks prematurely. Which of the following would provide the best postoperative analgesia in this patient?

a. Local infiltration and regular paracetamol.
b. Local infiltration and regular ibuprofen.
c. Local infiltration and morphine infusion.
d. Local infiltration and Oramorph.
e. Epidural analgesia.

22

Which of the following surgical procedures has the highest incidence of postoperative respiratory complications?

a. Abdominal aortic surgery.
b. Peripheral vascular surgery.
c. Abdominal surgery for bowel resection.
d. Neurosurgery.
e. Major head and neck surgery.

23

A 45-year-old female patient is scheduled for arthroscopy of the knee joint. During the pre-operative assessment she gives a history of sweating, dizziness and visual disturbances during the previous 2 months. During the previous week she had two such episodes lasting for a few minutes. She denies any history of diabetes or any other medical illness. She is not taking any regular medication. A random blood glucose level in the pre-operative clinic is 2.5mmol/L. The next most useful investigation in establishing the clinical diagnosis in this patient is:

a. Fasting blood glucose.
b. Urine ketone body levels.
c. Plasma insulin level.
d. CT scan of the abdomen.
e. MRI scan of the abdomen.

24 A 55-year-old woman presents to the emergency department with chest pain and shortness of breath. She was discharged from the hospital a week ago following fixation of a fractured ankle. On examination she has a respiratory rate of 30/minute, with a SpO_2 of 93% on 15L/min of oxygen. Her heart rate is 117 bpm and blood pressure is 110/46mm Hg. An ECG shows T-wave inversion in lead III. A bedside transthoracic echocardiogram suggests raised pulmonary artery pressure and right ventricular strain. Which of the following would be the most appropriate immediate management?

a.   Enoxaparin 1.5mg/kg administered subcutaneously.
b.   Urgent Doppler ultrasound of the leg veins.
c.   Alteplase 50mg intravenous bolus.
d.   Warfarin 10mg orally.
e.   Aspirin 300mg and clopidogrel 300mg orally.

25 A 45-year-old female patient with myasthenia gravis underwent a laparoscopic cholecystectomy. Her pre-operative medications included pyridostigmine 440mg and prednisolone 10mg per day. At induction vecuronium 0.05mg/kg was administered which resulted in loss of twitch responses to train of four stimulation. At the end of surgery neuromuscular blockade was reversed with neostigmine and glycopyrrolate. The trachea was extubated following confirmation of adequate reversal of blockade by both nerve stimulation and clinical signs. On transfer to recovery the patient develops muscle weakness and hypoventilation. Which of the following would be the most useful drug in deciding further management of this patient?

a.   Neostigmine.
b   Edrophonium.
c.   Pyridostigmine.
d.   Naloxone.
e.   Doxapram.

26 A 65-year-old male patient with severe COAD is scheduled for a total knee replacement. Routine pre-operative investigations reveal elevated blood levels of urea and creatinine. Which of the following is the most appropriate for postoperative pain relief?

a. Regular paracetamol and diclofenac sodium.
b. Intravenous morphine infusion.
c. Femoral nerve block and infiltration of the wound with lignocaine 0.5%.
d. Intrathecal morphine and regular paracetamol.
e. Combined femoral and sciatic nerve block and regular paracetamol.

27 A 25-year-old male patient is admitted to the intensive care unit following a thoracotomy for a stab injury of the chest. Six hours after surgery, following extubation, he suddenly starts complaining of shortness of breath. His core body temperature is 37°C, his pulse is irregular with a rate of 150 bpm, his respiratory rate is 25/minute and his blood pressure is 105/82mmHg. A 12-lead ECG shows atrial fibrillation with a ventricular rate of 160 per minute. Arterial blood gas shows a respiratory acidosis. On examination the patient is pale and sweaty. His JVP is 12mm Hg. There are no clinical signs of a pneumothorax or haemothorax. Which of the following would be the most appropriate immediate management in this situation?

a. Echocardiography and cardiology opinion.
b. Commence treatment with anticoagulants.
c. Start patient on digoxin and then consider electrical cardioversion.
d. Electrical cardioversion and start patient on aspirin and heparin.
e. Electrical cardioversion and consider cardiothoracic/cardiology opinion.

28 A 52-year-old man is scheduled for resection of an adrenal pheochromocytoma. His current treatment includes phenoxy-benzamine 40mg twice daily, commenced 10 days before. Over the past 3 days his heart rate has varied between 110-120 bpm. His blood pressure is 146/86mm Hg in the supine position and 110/68mm Hg when erect. The next step in his management should be:

a. Proceed with surgery.
b. Increase the dose of phenoxybenzamine.
c. Start propranolol 30mg twice daily.
d. Stop phenoxybenzamine and commence phentolamine instead.
e. Start enalapril 5mg once daily.

29 A 35-year-old female patient with a history of postoperative nausea and vomiting (PONV) is scheduled for a laser stapedectomy as a day-case procedure. Which of the following in the anaesthetic management is most likely to reduce PONV?

a. Avoiding neuromuscular blocking agents.
b. Premedication with anxiolytics.
c. Head-up tilt of 10-15°.
d. Total intravenous anaesthesia using propofol and remifentanil.
e. Induced hypotension.

30 A previously hypertensive patient is admitted to the intensive care unit after an emergency laparotomy for an anastomotic leak following an oesophagectomy. He was hypertensive and hypothermic in the recovery room, but after active warming, he is now normothermic, with a BP of 95/39mmHg, and heart rate of 110 bpm. His cardiac index is $3.2L/m^2$, PCWP is 3mmHg, SVR is $550dynes/cm/sec^{-5}$, and base excess is -7mmol/L. Over the last 2 hours, his total urine output is 35ml. Which of the following would be the most appropriate treatment to improve his renal function?

a. Administration of norepinephrine.
b. Administration of dobutamine.
c. Intravenous furosemide 40mg.
d. Intravenous mannitol 0.5g/kg.
e. Expansion circulating volume using a fluid challenge.

Set 6 answers

1   Answer: A. Mitral stenosis.

The normal area of the mitral valve orifice is about 4 to 6cm^2. When the mitral valve area is reduced below 2cm^2, there is an impediment to the flow of blood into the left ventricle, creating a pressure gradient across the mitral valve. The first heart sound is unusually loud and may be palpable (tapping apex beat) because of the increased force required to close the mitral valve. Stenosis of the mitral valve causes turbulent diastolic flow during diastole resulting in a mid-diastolic murmur, which is best heard at the apical region. Tricuspid stenosis causes a low rumbling diastolic murmur, which is best heard at the lower sternal border. Mitral regurgitation causes a pansystolic murmur. Aortic stenosis causes an ejection systolic murmur, which is best heard in the aortic area. Pulmonary stenosis results in a systolic murmur which is best heard in the pulmonary area. In mitral stenosis, enlargement of the left atrium produces straightening of the left border of the heart on a plain chest X-ray.

Further reading
1. Valvular heart disease. In: *Anesthesia and co-existing diseases*, 4th ed. Stoelting RK, Dierdorf S, Eds. Philadelphia, USA: Churchill Livingstone, 2002; Chapter 2: 33-5.

2   Answer: C. Intravenous phenytoin 18mg/kg, given over 30 minutes.

This child is suffering from status epilepticus; the priority is to stop the seizures. Initial supportive management includes ensuring a patent airway, administering 100% oxygen and assisting breathing. Rectal and buccal medications should only be administered in the pre-hospital setting. Senior help should also be sought promptly. If both benzodiazepines and paraldehyde have been given with no effect, the next line of therapy after intravenous access has been established is phenytoin. Although paracetamol is used to reduce the temperature in febrile convulsions, there is no evidence that antipyretics reduce the risk of subsequent febrile convulsions. In the above clinical scenario it may not be possible to administer medications orally.

Further reading

1. CG20 Epilepsy in adults and children: full guideline, appendix C (corrected). NICE clinical guidelines, October 2004.
2. Chapman MG, Smith M, Hirschz NP. Status epilepticus, review article. *Anaesthesia* 2001; 51: 648-59.
3. Appleton R, Choonara I, Martland T, *et al*. The treatment of convulsive status epilepticus in children. *Arch Dis Child* 2000; 83: 415-9.
4. El-Radhi AS, Barry W. Do antipyretics prevent febrile convulsions? *Arch Dis Child* 2003; 88: 641-2.
5. Young GM. Paediatric status epilepticus: treatment and medication. (http://emedicine.medscape.com/article/804189-treatment).

3   Answer: D. Citalopram.

This patient is exhibiting signs of serotoninergic syndrome commonly caused by overdose of selective serotonin reuptake blocking agents. Overdose of edrophonium will cause cholinergic syndrome (confusion, bradycardia, salivation, emesis and weakness). Overdose of benzodiazepines will result in respiratory depression, hypotension, hypothermia and hyporeflexia. Amitriptyline (tricyclic anti-depressant) overdose causes metabolic acidosis, a wide QRS complex, prolonged PR interval arrhythmias, convulsions and coma.

Further reading

1. http://www.toxbase.co.uk.
2. Mokhlesi B, Leiken JB, Murray P, *et al*. Adult toxicology in critical care: Part II Specific poisoning. *Chest* 2003; 123: 897-922.

4 Answer: C. Intravenous infusion of 0.9% saline solution.

This patient has developed hyponatraemia during the first week following head injury. Clinical examination and biochemical tests suggest that he is dehydrated, but the usual hypernatraemia seen with body water deficit is not apparent.

Hyponatraemia is common after traumatic brain injury and it is important to recognise the cause as the treatments differ significantly. The most common causes are, firstly, the syndrome of inappropriate anti-diuretic hormone secretion (SIADH) and, secondly, cerebral salt wasting syndrome (CSWS). Both are characterised by hyponatraemia but are differentiated by the intravascular volume status. This case has features suggestive of hypovolaemia and so is likely to be CSWS.

SIADH is a normo- or hyper-volaemic state caused by excessive re-absorption of free water. This causes haemodilution and is characterised by a low plasma osmolality with a normal or high urine osmolality. It is also important to assess the haemodynamic state; the key to the diagnosis of SIADH is the absence of clinical signs of dehydration. Treatment of SIADH is initially by restriction of water intake, followed by the administration of drugs such as demeclocycline which inhibits the renal response to ADH. It is also possible to use diuretics to increase fluid excretion, whilst supplementing sodium by other means.

CSWS is often misdiagnosed as SIADH and treated incorrectly. Biochemical criteria for CSWS include a low serum sodium with a high or normal plasma and urine osmolality. The key distinguishing feature is hypovolaemia. This should be assessed clinically; signs such as hypotension, low central venous pressure and dry mucous membranes are likely to be present. Examination of the fluid chart will often reveal a persistently negative fluid balance. Blood tests will show features of dehydration including a high urea and high haematocrit.

The pathophysiology of CSWS is still unclear, but is likely to involve the A-type and B-type natriuretic peptides. Treatment is by replacement of sodium and water, in most cases by the use of 0.9% saline solution.

Symptomatic hyponatraemia can be treated by the use of more concentrated saline solutions (1.8% or 3%) alongside diuretics to avoid circulatory overload.

Further reading
1. Bradshaw K, Smith M. Disorders of sodium balance after brain injury, *British Journal of Anaesthesia CEACCP* 2008; 8: 129-33.

5 Answer: D. Mechanical VTE prophylaxis and low-molecular-weight heparin continued for 28 days post-surgery.

According to NICE guidelines, the VTE risk of each patient should be assessed individually. This patient is at significantly increased risk of VTE as she has cancer, and is undergoing pelvic surgery with a period of immobility in bed postoperatively. Mechanical VTE prophylaxis and low-molecular-weight heparin should be prescribed and continued for 28 days post-surgery.

Further reading
1. CG92 Venous thromboembolism - reducing the risk. National Institute for Health and Clinical Excellence guidelines, 2010. (www.nice.org.uk).

6 Answer: C. Intravenous ketamine infusion.

This patient's pain is generalised in the stump area and is therefore unlikely to be neuroma-related pain. He did initially respond to opioid analgesics, but seemed to have developed acute tolerance to them. As he has a history of opioid addiction, acute tolerance to opioids is most likely. Administering epidural or intrathecal opioids is effective in patients who are responsive to opioid analgesia but cannot tolerate it due to side effects. Gabapentin may be useful in this patient but it is not available intravenously. Ketamine has been shown to reverse, at least partly reverse, acute opioid tolerance in doses that are not large enough to provide a direct antinociceptive effect. Therefore, intravenous infusion in the dose range of 10 to 20mg/hour is likely to be the most effective.

Further reading

1. Yamauchi M, Asano M, Watanabe M, *et al.* Continuous low-dose ketamine improves the analgesic effects of fentanyl patient-controlled analgesia after cervical spine surgery. *Anesth Analg* 2008; 107: 1041-4.

7   Answer: B. Cerebral oedema.

Cerebral oedema occurs in up to 1% of all paediatric diabetic ketoacidosis (DKA). It is the most common cause of mortality in children with DKA, accounting for 60-90% of all paediatric DKA deaths. Other causes of mortality include hypokalaemia and hyperkalaemia with associated arrhythmias, sepsis, aspiration pneumonia, acute pancreatitis, intracranial venous thrombosis and rhabdomyolysis.

Further reading

1. Steel S, Tibby SM. Paediatric diabetic ketoacidosis. *British Journal of Anaesthesia CEACCP* 2009; 9: 194-9.

8   Answer: D. Autoimmune hypothyroidism.

The clinical features are suggestive of hypothyroidism. Elevated TSH levels together with low T3 and T4 levels suggest that she is experiencing primary hypothyroidism. Primary hypothyroidism is due to intrinsic thyroid gland failure. The most common cause is autoimmune hypothyroidism. It is six times more common in females. Other causes of primary hypothyroidism include irradiation, thyroid surgery and iodine deficiency or excess.

Secondary hypothyroidism is due to inadequate levels of TSH with a normal thyroid gland. This can be due to pituitary failure or pituitary surgery. All levels of TSH, T3 and T4 will be low. Hypothalamic failure results in tertiary hypothyroidism, due to low levels of TRH.

Further reading

1. Farling PA. Thyroid disease. *British Journal of Anaesthesia* 2000; 85: 15-28.

2. Howlett TA. Endocrine disease. In: *Clinical medicine*, 6th ed. Kumar P, Clark M. Philadelphia, USA: Elsevier Saunders, 2005; Chapter 18: 1073-80.

9 Answer: E. *Herpes simplex* virus.

The results of CSF analysis suggest viral meningitis. Common viruses that can cause meningitis include arbovirus, cytomegalovirus and the *Herpes simplex* virus. This patient should be treated with I.V. acyclovir (10mg/kg 8- hourly). CSF findings in early bacterial meningitis and partially treated bacterial meningitis may be similar to those found with viral meningitis. Viral meningitis is also known as aseptic meningitis due to the inability to isolate pathogens in CSF. In viral meningitis, the CSF biochemistry is likely to reveal low protein and an elevated white cell count, predominantly monocytes (lymphocytes). The CSF biochemistry in meningitis is shown in Table 1.

Table 1. CSF biochemistry in meningitis.

Parameter	Normal value	Bacterial meningitis	Viral meningitis
WCC	$<5/mm^3$	$>1000/mm^3$	$<1000/mm^3$
Glucose	3.3-4.4mmol/L	<2/3 plasma level	>2/3 plasma level
Protein	0.2-0.4g/L	0.5-2g/L	0.4-0.8g/L

Further reading
1. Steiner I, Budka H, Chaudhuri A, *et al*. Viral encephalitis: a review of diagnostic methods and guidelines for management. *European Journal of Neurology* 2005; 12: 331-45.
2. Van de Beek D, de Gans J, Tunkel AR, *et al*. Community-acquired bacterial meningitis in adults. *N Engl J Med* 2006; 354: 44-53.

10 Answer: D. Obliteration of the third ventricle.

All of the above findings on the CT scan are associated with a poor prognosis. Obliteration of the third ventricle and midline shift are, however, the strongest predictors of mortality at 14 days.

Further reading
1. The MRC CRASH Trial Collaborators. Predicting outcome after traumatic brain injury: practical prognostic models based on a large cohort of international patients. *BMJ* 2008; 336: 425-9.

11 Answer: D. Gabapentin.

This patient is suffering from post-amputation limb pain. Following amputation, the incidence of chronic pain is very high. There are three types of pain problems which can occur after amputation. These are stump pain, neuroma pain or phantom limb pain. Stump pain usually occurs as a result of infection, scar tissue or bony stump irritation due to inadequate padding by muscle. Neuroma pain is due to abnormal outgrowth of the nerve from the cut end. It is generally localised pain and elicited by touch or pressure over the neuroma. Phantom limb pain is pain experienced in the missing part of the limb. One of the proposed theories is that when a limb is amputated many severed nerve endings outgrow abnormally and/or become inflamed and send anomalous signals to the brain. These signals are thought to be interpreted by the brain as pain. At times, the patient may feel as if they are gesturing, feel itches, twitch, or even feel as if they are trying to pick things up.

This particular patient has phantom limb pain and therefore gabapentin would be the most appropriate initial therapy. If this fails, intervention therapy or, more recently recommended, image-guided therapy could be considered. Image-guided therapy is a novel treatment for phantom limb pain. Through the use of artificial visual feedback (mirror box) it becomes possible for the patient to 'move' the phantom limb, and to unclench it from potentially painful positions. Repeated training in some subjects has led to long-term improvement.

Further reading

1. Halbert J, Crotty M, Cameron ID. Evidence for the optimal management of acute and chronic phantom pain: a systematic review. *Clin J Pain* 2002; 18: 84-92.

12 Answer: A. Axillary petechiae.

The diagnosis of fat embolism is usually made on the basis of clinical findings. The major criteria are based on the classic triad of respiratory insufficiency, neurological impairment and a petechial rash. Although a petechial rash is present in only 20-50% of cases, it is considered pathognomonic of fat embolism. To establish the diagnosis of fat embolism syndrome, at least one major and four minor criteria must be present.

Major criteria include:

- Axillary or sub-conjunctival petechiae.
- Hypoxaemia PaO_2 <60mm Hg.
- Central nervous system depression disproportionate to the hypoxaemia.
- Pulmonary oedema.

Minor criteria include:

- Tachycardia.
- Pyrexia.
- The presence of fat in the urine.
- The presence of retinal emboli.
- Increased ESR.

Further reading

1. Gupta A, Reilly CS. Fat embolism. *British Journal of Anaesthesia CEACCP* 2007; 7: 148-51.

13 Answer: E. Baclofen.

The symptoms described in the postoperative period are those due to acute withdrawal of baclofen. The majority of patients with cerebral palsy are likely to be taking a combination of anti-epileptics, antidepressants, baclofen and analgesics. As this patient developed postoperative nausea and vomiting she may have omitted her regular oral baclofen during the postoperative period as well. Sudden cessation of baclofen may result in acute withdrawal symptoms such as disorientation, painful muscle spasms, dystonia, seizures, bradycardia and hypotension.

Baclofen is a $GABA_A$ receptor agonist, which acts as an inhibitory neurotransmitter in the central nervous system. It can be given orally or intrathecally through a subcutaneously implanted continuous infusion device. Ondansetron has very mild side effects on I.V. administration, such as headache, a sensation of warmth, occasional visual disturbances and transient dizziness.

Further reading

1. Prosser DP, Sharma N. Cerebral palsy and anaesthesia. *British Journal of Anaesthesia CEACCP* 2001; 10: 72-6.

14 Answer: C. Activated charcoal.

Activated charcoal is used in the management of many orally ingested toxins due to its adsorptive capacity. It is effective if administered within the first hour of ingestion. A recent Cochrane review concluded that activated charcoal is more effective than gastric lavage or ipecac-induced emesis in preventing absorption of paracetamol. N-acetyl cysteine and methionine are used in the treatment of paracetamol overdose but do not reduce the absorption of paracetamol.

Further reading

1. Ward W, Sair M. Oral poisoning: an update. *British Journal of Anaesthesia CEACCP* 2010; 10: 6-11.

15 Answer: B. Oxygen and intravenous Hartmann's solution.

This man may have sickle cell disease (SCD), an inherited haemoglobinopathy resulting from a mutation in chromosome 11 which leads to the substitution of valine for glutamate at position 6 of the beta Hb chain, producing HbS. HbS precipitates in the deoxygenated form and may lead to sickling of the red blood cell. Sickling of red blood cells is exacerbated by stasis, cold, dehydration and sepsis. Acute 'crises' are most often vaso-occlusive, presenting with an acute abdomen, pulmonary infarction, bone infarction, stroke and priapism. Aplastic crises lead to marrow shutdown usually caused by parvovirus B19, while sequestration crises are seen usually in children with massive pooling of red cells in the spleen. Patients are usually anaemic (Hb 6-9g/dL) and develop progressive organ damage including asplenism, renal impairment, cardiomegaly, pulmonary hypertension, retinal damage and cerebrovascular disease. Heterozygotes (HbAS) produce normal Hb and about 30-40% HbS. Diagnosis is by electrophoresis which distinguishes type and quantity of different haemoglobins. The Sickledex test is a screening test which can rapidly detect the presence of HbS if greater than 10%, and is positive in both disease and trait. The blood film in SCD will usually show anaemia with reticulocytosis, target and sickle cells, whereas it is often normal in trait.

In this scenario, the acute abdomen may represent a crisis, therefore immediate measures should include rehydration and oxygen as well as analgesia. The need for surgery may then be reassessed in light of the response and Sickledex results. If surgery is required, it may be advised to transfuse to an Hb of >10g/dL following advice from a haematologist.

Further reading

1. Haemoglobinopathy and sickle cell disease. *British Journal of Anaesthesia CEACCP* 2010; 10: 24-7.

16 Answer: B. Penile block and regular paracetamol and ibuprofen.

Postoperative pain after circumcision is usually well controlled using regular paracetamol and ibuprofen. It is a simple regime, which can safely be administered at home. Caudal block is effective in providing analgesia after circumcision and is commonly used. However, 10ml of 0.5% bupivacaine (50mg) in this child will exceed the maximum dose and is likely to cause urinary retention and leg weakness. The dose of ketamine for caudal use is in the range of 0.5 to 1mg/kg and the higher dose is likely to cause unpleasant CNS side effects. Regular Oramorph is rarely needed for circumcision and has side effects such as nausea, vomiting and sedation. Penile block with regular paracetamol and ibuprofen would be safe and effective pain relief in this patient.

Further reading
1. Joyce BA, Keck JF, Gerkensmeyer J. Evaluation of pain management interventions for neonatal circumcision pain. *Journal of Pediatric Health Care* 2001; 15: 105-14.

17 Answer: D. Insertion of an automatic implantable cardioverter defibrillator (AICD).

The aim of treatment is to prevent sudden death from fatal arrhythmias such as Torsades de Pointes. Beta-blockers are the first line in the treatment of long QT syndrome (LQTS), but they may be ineffective in about 25% of patients. Anti-bradycardia pacing is indicated in patients with bradycardia and pauses. An AICD is the treatment of choice when the initial presentation is a cardiac arrest, in symptomatic patients despite beta-blockers, and in patients with documented arrhythmia despite beta-blockers.

Long QT syndrome complicated by Torsades de Pointes can be treated with intravenous magnesium sulphate. Amiodarone is not effective in preventing arrhythmias associated with long QT syndrome.

Further reading

1. Al-Refai A, Gunka V, Douglas J. Spinal anaesthesia for Caesarean section in a parturient with long QT syndrome. *Canadian Journal of Anaesthesia* 2004; 51: 993-6.
2. Drake E, Preston R, Douglas J. Brief review: anaesthetic implications of long QT syndrome in pregnancy. *Canadian Journal of Anaesthesia* 2007; 54: 561-72.

18 Answer: D. Transfusion-related acute lung injury (TRALI)

Since the clinical deterioration occurred following blood transfusion, it is most likely to be related to the blood transfusion. The possibility of TRALI should be considered in any patient developing hypoxaemia and pulmonary oedema within a few hours of transfusion of any blood product or plasma derivative containing plasma.

TRALI is a form of acute respiratory distress syndrome due to transfusion of blood products containing plasma. The onset is usually within the first 6 hours, though it can occur up to 24 hours after transfusion. The mechanism of TRALI involves activation of recipient leucocytes by donor anti-leucocyte antibodies.

Cardiogenic shock can occur secondary to a myocardial event in a patient with significant cardiovascular disease. Similarly, volume overload may occur in patients with pre-existing cardiorespiratory disease.

Further reading

1. Teague G, Hughes A, Gaylard D. Transfusion-related acute lung injury. *Anesthesia Intensive Care* 2005; 33: 124-7.
2. Rajan GR. Severe transfusion-related acute lung injury in the intensive care unit secondary to transfusion of fresh frozen plasma. *Anaesthesia Intensive Care* 2005; 33: 400-2.

19   Answer: A. Septicaemia.

Oesophagectomy is associated with multiple potential complications, including oesophageal anastomotic leak, chest infection, deep vein thrombosis, myocardial infarction, gastric necrosis, and prolonged ileus. The postoperative mortality rate associated with oesophagectomy ranges from 5% to 13%. The most common causes of morbidity and mortality are cardiopulmonary complications. The rise in temperature, hypotension, tachycardia, and a low CVP indicate sepsis as the most likely cause of his collapse. In severe dehydration or haemorrhage or myocardial infarction, the patient's temperature is likely to be normal. In cardiac tamponade, the CVP will be high.

Further reading

1. Nozoe T, Kimura Y, Ishida M, *et al.* Correlation of pre-operative nutritional condition with postoperative complications in surgical treatment for oesophageal carcinoma. *Eur J Surg Oncol* 2002; 28: 396-400.

20   Answer: E. ECG.

The history is suggestive of myotonia dystrophica. It is a multisystem disease inherited as an autosomal dominant trait. Patients usually present at the age of 15-35 years. Increased muscle tone on exercise, respiratory muscle weakness, cataracts, testicular atrophy, frontal balding, obstructive sleep apnoea, and cardiomyopathy are associated features. First-degree heart block is a common finding on the ECG. Sudden death can occur due to complete heart block. Up to 20% of patients may have evidence of mitral valve prolapse on echocardiography.

Although ultrasound of the gall bladder is a useful investigation to evaluate the presence of gall stones, it is more relevant to surgical management. Electromyography is not helpful in this situation but may be useful in the diagnosis of myasthenia gravis.

Anaesthetic implications in these patients include poor cardiorespiratory reserve, delayed gastric emptying, and increased sensitivity to I.V.

anaesthetics and non-depolarising agents. Suxamethonium may cause prolonged muscle contraction.

Further reading
1. Russell SH, Hirsch P. Anaesthesia and myotonia, review article. *British Journal of Anaesthesia* 1994; 72: 210-6
2. Myotonic dystrophy In: *Anesthesia and co-existing disease*, 4th ed. Stoelting RK, Dierdorf SF, Eds. Philadelphia, USA: Churchill Livingstone, 2002; 519-20.

21 Answer: A. Local infiltration and regular paracetamol.

The surgical procedure of pyloromyotomy involves a small sub-costal incision and pain following this can be managed by local infiltration and regular paracetamol. NSAIDs should be avoided below the age of 6 months due to their effect on pulmonary circulation. Opioids are generally avoided below the age of 6 months due to their side effects. There is a risk of postoperative apnoea in neonates and the biochemical changes associated with pyloric stenosis can also predispose to opioid-induced postoperative respiratory depression.

Further reading
1. Fell D, Chelliah S. Infantile pyloric stenosis. *British Journal of Anaesthesia CEPD Reviews* 2001; 1: 85-8.

22 Answer: A. Abdominal aortic surgery.

The risk of overall postoperative respiratory complications is about 25% with open abdominal aortic surgery. The incidence of postoperative pneumonia is higher with abdominal aortic surgery compared to thoracic surgery (odds ratio 4.3 versus 3.9).

Endovascular repair is associated with a much lower risk of postoperative pneumonia as compared to an open procedure.

Further reading
1. Moppett IK. Respiratory risk. In: *Consent, benefit, and risk in anaesthetic practice*. Hardmann JG, Moppett IK, Aitkenhead AR, Eds. Oxford: Oxford University Press, 2009; Chapter 12: 173-87.

23 Answer: C. Plasma insulin level.

The possible diagnosis in this patient is insulinoma; this is an insulin-secreting tumour arising from the islet cells of the pancreas. It may secrete insulin in short bursts, causing wide fluctuations in the blood levels. About 90% of insulinomas are benign, and 10% are malignant. Roughly 10% of patients have multiple insulinomas.

The diagnosis is based mainly on the presence of inappropriately high levels of insulin (>10 micro units), a low plasma glucose (<2.5mmol/L), and plasma c-peptide levels >2.5ng during overnight or supervised fasting for 72 hours.

Imaging studies such as an ultrasound scan, a CT scan and an MRI scan are only indicated once the biochemical tests confirm the diagnosis, because the majority of tumours are smaller than 2cm, which are difficult to detect using imaging studies.

Further reading
1. Ali AZ, Radebold K. Insulinoma. (http://emedicine.medscape.com/article/283039-diagnosis).

24 Answer: A. Enoxaparin 1.5mg/kg administered subcutaneously.

The most likely diagnosis is pulmonary embolism (PE). The patient is relatively stable but demonstrates signs of right heart strain on the ECG and echocardiogram. Current evidence suggests that the risks of thrombolysis (such as GI bleed, haemorrhagic stroke) outweigh the benefits unless there is significant haemodynamic instability or cardiac arrest. It is therefore not indicated in this case.

Initial treatment should be with a 'treatment-dose' low-molecular-weight heparin, and this should be continued while long-term anticoagulation is established. Warfarin is ineffective for 2-3 days following the start of therapy and so is not the correct initial treatment.

The most likely source of embolus is a vein in the leg that has recently been treated for the fracture. If there are clinical signs of DVT then a Doppler ultrasound should be arranged, but treatment should be started in the meantime. If a DVT is not found then a CT pulmonary angiogram will be necessary to confirm the diagnosis, but again this should not delay treatment.

Further reading
1. Van Beek EJR, Elliot CA, Kiely DG. Diagnosis and initial treatment of patients with suspected pulmonary thromboembolism. *British Journal of Anaesthesia CEACCP* 2009; 9: 119-24.

25 Answer: B. Edrophonium.

The likely cause for muscle weakness and hypoventilation in this patient is either a cholinergic crisis or a myasthenic crisis. Both can result in muscle weakness. A cholinergic crisis occurs as a result of excessive acetylcholine, due to an excessive dose of anticholinesterase. In a cholinergic crisis, the pupils are constricted, whereas in a myasthenic crisis they are dilated. In a myasthenic crisis a small dose of edrophonium improves muscle strength; in a cholinergic crisis it does not improve muscle weakness. A myasthenic crisis should be treated with pyridostigmine. Any further doses of neostigmine should be used cautiously to avoid a cholinergic crisis. Doxapram is a respiratory stimulant and naloxone reverses opioid-induced respiratory depression.

Further reading
1. Myasthenic syndrome. In: *Anesthesia and co-existing diseases*, 4th ed. Stoelting RK, Dierdorf S, Eds. Philadelphia, USA: Churchill Livingstone, 2002; Chapter 26: 527-8.
2. Abel M. Myasthenia gravis. In: *Clinical cases in anaesthesia*, 3rd ed. Reed AP, Yudkowitz FS, Eds. Philadelphia, USA: Elsevier Churchill Livingstone, 2005; Case 27: 137-42.

26 Answer: E. Combined femoral and sciatic nerve block and regular paracetamol.

A combined femoral and sciatic nerve block is effective in providing adequate postoperative analgesia for up to 24 hours in the postoperative period. Both systemic and intrathecal opioids can cause respiratory depression and this risk is increased in a patient with severe COAD. Although NSAIDs are generally recommended for postoperative analgesia, they would be inappropriate in a patient with deranged renal function.

Further reading

1. Fischer HBJ, Simanski CJP, Sharp C. A procedure-specific systematic review and consensus recommendations for post-operative analgesia following total knee arthroplasty. *Anaesthesia* 2008; 63: 1105-23.

27 Answer: E. Electrical cardioversion and consider cardiothoracic/cardiology opinion.

Unless contraindicated, a rhythm-control strategy should be the initial management option for the treatment of postoperative atrial fibrillation (AF) following cardiothoracic surgery. Any underlying electrolyte imbalance should be corrected and prophylaxis with anti-thrombotic therapy (in consultation with cardiology) should be considered.

In general, the evidence suggests that combined therapeutic anticoagulation with antiplatelet therapy does not reduce the incidence of stroke or thrombo-embolism when compared to therapeutic anticoagulation alone, and it may increase the incidence of bleeding. Preloading with anti-arrhythmic drugs prior to electrical cardioversion does not appear to have any long-term efficacy in maintaining sinus rhythm.

Further reading

1. NICE guidelines for the management of atrial fibrillation, June 2006.

28 Answer: C. Start propranolol 30mg twice daily.

Adequate pre-operative preparation is essential prior to surgery in order to reduce mortality and morbidity. Alpha-blockade with oral phenoxybenzamine is the treatment of choice for pheochromocytoma. It should be started at 10mg per day and gradually increased until postural hypotension develops. As the alpha-blockade is established, the intravascular volume expands and tachycardia may develop which should be treated with adequate hydration. Beta-blockade can be used to treat associated tachycardia. Beta-blockers should not be started until adequate alpha-blockade is established, as an unopposed alpha-adrenergic effect may precipitate a hypertensive crisis and cardiac failure.

This patient has adequate alpha-blockade as indicated by his postural hypotension. His tachycardia should be treated with propranolol. Both drugs should be continued. Enalapril is an angiotensin-converting enzyme inhibitor and is not usually used in the management of pheochromocytoma.

Further reading

1. Prys-Roberts C. Phaeochromocytoma - recent progress in its management. *British Journal of Anaesthesia* 2000; 85: 44-57.
2. Pace N, Buttigieg M. Phaeochromocytoma. *British Journal of Anaesthesia CEPD review* 2003; 3: 20-3.
3. Malhotra V, Garland TA. Pheochromocytoma. In: *Decision making in anesthesiology - an algorithmic approach*, 3rd ed. Bready LL, Mullins RM, Noorily SH, Smith RB, Eds. Missouri, USA: Mosby, 180-1.

29 Answer: D. Total intravenous anaesthesia using propofol and remifentanil.

Middle ear surgery is associated with a high incidence of PONV. The reported incidence is as high as 80% in adults without anti-emetic prophylaxis. The use of total intravenous anaesthesia using propofol is a popular technique for middle ear surgery, as a reduced incidence of PONV, reduced bleeding and better operating conditions have been observed.

There is no contraindication to the use of neuromuscular blocking agents at induction of anaesthesia, though avoiding further doses of neuromuscular blocking agents facilitates monitoring of the facial nerve using a nerve stimulator. This patient may be very anxious due to the previous experience of nausea and vomiting, so premedication with benzodiazepines may be helpful in reducing the anxiety. Induced hypotension and a slight head-up tilt reduces bleeding at the surgical site.

Further reading

1. Herlich A. Tympanomastoidectomy. In: *Clinical cases in anaesthesia*, 3rd ed. Reed AP, Yudkowitz FS, Eds. Philadelphia, USA: Elsevier Churchill Livingstone, 2005; Case 45: 243-5.

30 Answer: E. Expansion circulating volume using a fluid challenge.

This patient has low systemic vascular resistance (SVR) and hypovolaemia as indicated by the low PCWP. Clinical signs also indicate that the patient is volume depleted probably due to sequestration of the fluid in the peritoneal cavity and increased capillary permeability due to sepsis. Mannitol will increase urine output but will worsen the hypovolaemia. Furosemide can cause a diuresis but will not improve renal function. Administration of dobutamine would be appropriate if the urine output does not improve despite restoration of the circulating volume.

Further reading

1. Carcillo JA, Tasker RC. Fluid resuscitation of hypovolemic shock: acute medicine's great triumph for children. *Intensive Care Med* 2006; 32: 958-61.
2. Sturm JA, Wisner DH. Fluid resuscitation of hypovolaemia. *Intensive Care Medicine* 1985; 11: 227-30.